MW01169823

Blood Pressure

Blood Pressure Solution: The Step-By-Step Guide to Lowering High Blood Pressure the Natural Way in 30 Days!

Natural Remedies to Reduce Hypertension Without Medication

Eva Coleman

ISBN: 1533167850
ISBN-13: 978-1533167859

Contents

FREE BLOOD PRESSURE SOLUTION AUDIOBOOK

Find this on the final page of the book.

not affiliated with this document.

This book is not intended as a substitute for the medical advice of physicians. The reader should regularly consult a physician in matters relating to his/her health and particularly with respect to any symptoms that may require diagnosis or medical attention.

Foreword

According to the World Health Organization, high blood pressure or hypertension, affects approximately 22% of adults worldwide. In the United States alone, around **70% of adults have high or raised blood pressure** – that is one in every three American adults.

Generally speaking, the higher the blood pressure, the higher the risk of damage to the heart and the blood vessels. High blood pressure is a chronic disease. If left untreated, hypertension can cause an array of health problems, including heart attack, cardiomegaly (an abnormal enlargement of the heart), heart failure, kidney failure, blindness, and cognitive impairment.

Thankfully, high blood pressure is treatable and taking preventative measures to control your blood pressure is the best way to protect your health. After all, prevention is better than cure and there is a lot that you can do to prevent and control your blood pressure. In most cases, lifestyle changes are completely effective in controlling blood pressure. We will cover all of the different natural hypertension prevention strategies available to you in *Section 3* of this guide. With an emphasis on prevention, we will provide you with all of the knowledge and strategies you need to prevent high blood pressure – permanently! If you already have high blood pressure, the same methods can also be used to control and lower your blood pressure to a healthy level.

By the end of this guide, you will:

- Understand the causes of high blood pressure and how high blood pressure affects your body and health.
- Know how to measure your own blood pressure!
- Be aware of the risk factors associated with high blood pressure.
- Know how to control and reduce your blood pressure.
- Know how to incorporate lifestyle changes that can lower your blood pressure.
- Know how to treat high blood pressure once you have been diagnosed.
- Be able to develop a nutritious and balanced diet plan.
- Be able to develop an exercise program, lose weight and stay healthy.
- Know how to practice relaxation and manage stress healthily.
- Know what substances and medications to avoid.
- Be able to reduce your blood pressure and improve your long-term health, happiness and wellbeing.

The ultimate goal of this guide is for you to gain a solid understanding of antihypertensive therapies that have been proven to control blood pressure. This is presented to you in clear language and easy-to-understand steps - allowing and empowering you take complete control of your health.

Congratulations on taking this first step to a better and healthier life!

Best wishes,

Eva Coleman

Section 1: Blood Pressure Explained

High blood pressure or hypertension, often referred to as the 'silent killer', is typically asymptomatic – meaning no symptoms are shown. Some people with high blood pressure will experience symptoms, including chest pain, dizziness, headaches, shortness of breath, palpitations, and heart and nose bleeds. Most people however, will experience no symptoms as all – until the damage has been done, which is often after several years of living with high blood pressure.

The first step to preventing and managing high blood pressure is to *understand* high blood pressure, its causes, effects, and long-term consequences. All of this will be covered in this section. If you already have high blood pressure, it is important to control and continuously monitor your blood pressure. Because of this, we will discuss how to monitor your own blood pressure at home in **subsection 4**. We will cover everything you need to know and take into account in order to create a successful blood pressure treatment plan – all without any prescription medications!

1. *Understanding High Blood Pressure and Blood Pressure Readings*

Blood pressure is a measurement of the force of blood which pushes against the walls of the arteries. The arteries are the large blood vessels that carry blood from the heart muscle to all of the other organs and muscles inside the body. As the blood is transported around the body, it pushes against the inside of the artery walls. The force of this 'push' is what we measure as blood pressure.

High blood pressure or hypertension is a medical condition in which the arteries are persistently subjected to an elevated blood pressure. This increased pressure is caused by a rise in the force of blood pushing against the walls of the arteries. The increased pressure can be caused by the arteries becoming thicker or hardening due to a build-up of plaque. Thicker artery walls mean that there is less space for the blood to flow through the arteries. This thickening (or narrowing of the artery) results in abnormal blood flow whereby the blood pushes harder against the walls of the arteries. This raises the blood pressure.

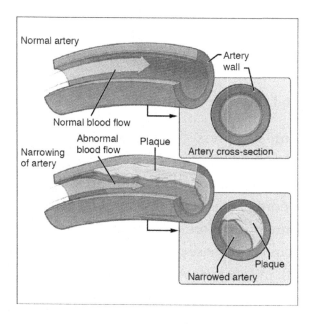

The higher the pressure, the greater the stress the arteries are under, and the more difficult it is for the heart to pump and deliver blood to the body. When blood pressure is high, this places stress on the body, which in turn can cause damage to the heart, kidneys, brain, and eyes.

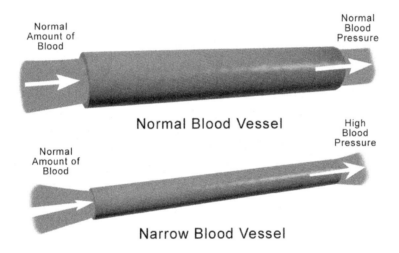

Normal Amount of Blood

Normal Blood Pressure

Normal Blood Vessel

Normal Amount of Blood

High Blood Pressure

Narrow Blood Vessel

How Is Blood Pressure Measured?

Blood pressure is expressed using two numbers - the systolic pressure (as the heart beats) over the diastolic pressure (as the heart relaxes). The normal systolic pressure is 120 mm Hg and the normal diastolic pressure is 80 mm Hg. Normal blood pressure is therefore written as 120 over 80, or 120/80. We will discuss how these numbers are determined in further depth in *subsection 4*, where we cover how blood pressure is measured.

Your pulse pressure is the difference between the systolic pressure reading and the diastolic pressure reading. Pulse pressure indicates the force that your heart muscle generates each time it contracts. Therefore, provided your blood pressure is normal, that is a reading of 120/80 mm Hg, then your pulse pressure is 40 (120 - 80 = 40).

As per the JNC7 report and guidelines, the following are the current blood pressure categories and their respective systolic and diastolic pressure values:

Category	Systolic Pressure	Diastolic Pressure
Optimal	115 or less	75 or less
Normal	120 or less	80 or less
Prehypertension	121 – 139	81 – 89
Stage 1 Hypertension	140 – 159	90 – 99
Stage 2 Hypertension	160 or more	100 or more

Blood pressure is considered to be high when the systolic blood pressure is equal to or greater than 140 mm Hg and/or the diastolic blood pressure is equal to or greater than 90 mm Hg (= 140/90). If any one value (systolic or diastolic) is in one of the elevated blood pressure categories, the patient is considered to be in that specific 'stage' of high blood pressure.

Your blood pressure goal should be 120/80, or even better, 115/75.

2. *The Causes, Types and Stages of High Blood Pressure*

There are some unchangeable factors as well as some changeable factors that contribute to high blood pressure.

In general, unchangeable factors that can be the root cause of high blood pressure include age, sex, ethnicity, family history and the person's medical history. Changeable factors which also have an impact on high blood pressure include diet, exercise routine, and stress management.

Essential Hypertension (Primary Blood Pressure)

Essential hypertension, also referred to as primary high blood pressure, is where the exact cause of the high blood pressure is unknown. The causes of essential hypertension can be genetic, due to aging, or influenced by environmental factors.

Some of the most common environmental factors thought to have impacted on high blood pressure include:

- Depression.
- Excess caffeine consumption.
- High salt intake – this raises the blood pressure in salt sensitive individuals.
- Lack of physical activity.
- Obesity.

- Stress.

Secondary Hypertension

Secondary high blood pressure is blood pressure resulting from a disease. To put it differently, secondary hypertension is high blood pressure where there is an identifiable cause.

Secondary causes/conditions that can cause high blood pressure include but are not limited to:

- Acromegaly – abnormal enlargement or growth of the hands, feet, and face.
- Coarctation (narrowing) of the aorta.
- Conn's syndrome.
- Cushing's syndrome.
- Hyperaldosteronism – a condition of excessive secretion of aldosterone leading to high blood pressure and low potassium levels.
- Hyperthyroidism – a condition characterized by a rapid heartbeat caused by the abnormal over-activity of a thyroid gland or Hypothyroidism – a condition where the activity of the thyroid gland is abnormally low.
- Kidney disease – kidney disease is the most common secondary cause of high blood pressure.
- Obesity.
- Pheochromocytoma – tumor of the adrenal medulla.
- Pregnancy - high blood pressure during pregnancy is explained in *Section 2, subsection 4.*

- Sleep apnea.

One of the most effective ways in which you can gain an understanding of your current health is to routinely measure your blood pressure using a home monitoring device. How to go about doing this will be covered later on in this section.

Different Stages of High Blood Pressure:

- **Prehypertension:** Individuals considered to fall under the prehypertension classification are strongly encouraged to adapt health-promoting lifestyle changes and modifications.
- **Stage 1 Hypertension:** During this stage, defined by a constriction of arteries or an increase in blood volume, high blood pressure is reversible.
- **Stage 2 Hypertension:** During this stage, characterized by the permanent thickening of the blood vessels, high blood pressure is irreversible without the use of medication.
- **Stage 3 Hypertension:** This is a hypertensive emergency.

Blood Pressure Category	Systolic (mm Hg)		Diastolic (mm Hg)
Normal	Less than 120	And	Less than 80
Prehypertension	120 – 139	Or	80 – 90
High Blood Pressure Stage 1	140 – 159	Or	90 – 99
High Blood Pressure Stage 2	160 or higher	Or	100 or higher
Hypertensive Crisis (Emergency Care Needed)	180 or higher	Or	110 or higher

3. *Why is High Blood Pressure Dangerous?*

High blood pressure is incredibly dangerous due to the associated health risks, including heart disease, blindness, cognitive impairment, and damage to the brain, kidneys, and blood vessels. If left uncontrolled and untreated, high blood pressure can lead to an enlargement of the heart, heart attack, and eventually to heart failure and death.

High blood pressure is in fact the most significant preventable cause of stroke and heart disease around the world.

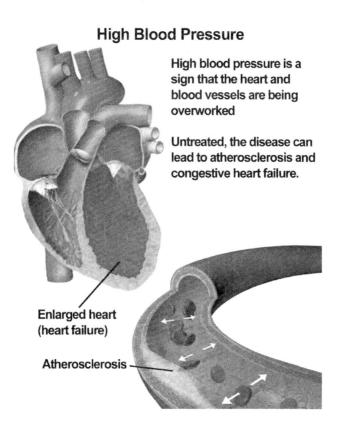

High Blood Pressure

High blood pressure is a sign that the heart and blood vessels are being overworked

Untreated, the disease can lead to atherosclerosis and congestive heart failure.

Enlarged heart (heart failure)

Atherosclerosis

The consequences of chronic high blood pressure can be worsened by other factors that increase the likeliness of stroke, heart attack and kidney failure. These include alcohol abuse, tobacco use, persistent stress, obesity, high cholesterol, diabetes mellitus, an unhealthy diet, and a general lack of physical activity. The best thing to do is not worry if any of these habits apply to you and your current lifestyle. We will discuss these in further detail and how to tackle them in *Section 3* of this guide.

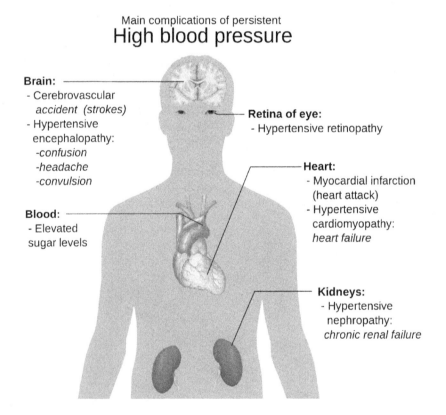

Main complications of persistent
High blood pressure

Brain:
- Cerebrovascular
  accident (strokes)
- Hypertensive
  encephalopathy:
  -confusion
  -headache
  -convulsion

Retina of eye:
- Hypertensive retinopathy

Heart:
- Myocardial infarction
  (heart attack)
- Hypertensive
  cardiomyopathy:
  heart failure

Blood:
- Elevated
  sugar levels

Kidneys:
- Hypertensive
  nephropathy:
  chronic renal failure

4. *How to Accurately Test Your Blood Pressure*

Blood pressure self-measurements are an ideal way to give you a better understanding of your blood pressure and your health. If your blood pressure is normal, it will suffice to have your blood pressure checked during routine check-ups. If you have been diagnosed with hypertension, measuring your blood pressure at home is an ideal way to track your progress and also give you a source of motivation!

The instrument used for measuring blood pressure is called a *sphygmomanometer.* Other easier terms to describe this device include blood measure meter, blood measure monitor, and blood measure gauge.

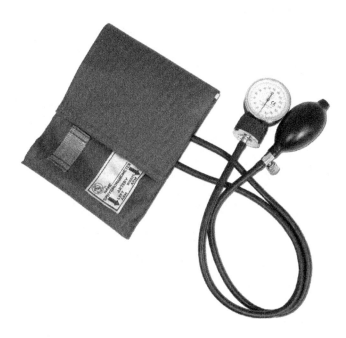

The blood pressure monitor in the above picture is called an **'aneroid blood pressure gauge'**, which is inexpensive to buy and easy to use. It is important to note though that if you're using an aneroid blood pressure gauge at home, it is important to validate and calibrate your instrument at your health clinic on a regular basis. This verification should be done at least every 6 months in order to ensure accuracy of your blood pressure readings.

You will also need a stethoscope which is a medical instrument that allows you to listen to various sounds inside the body. The stethoscope is composed of ear pieces and a bell, which is the point of contact.

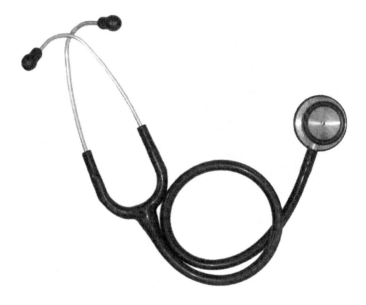

In order to get an accurate blood pressure reading, follow the steps below:

Before taking your blood pressure:

- **Do not exercise, eat, smoke, drink alcohol or coffee for at least 15 minutes prior to taking your blood pressure.** This is because all of these factors can have an impact on your blood pressure reading.
- **Make sure you use a properly sized blood pressure cuff.** The length of the bladder of the cuff should be at least 80% of the circumference of your upper arm. Use small cuffs on children and large cuffs if you are overweight or muscular.
- **Get the posture right!** Sit down with your arm and back supported. Your elbow should be supported at around the same level of your heart, e.g. on a table next to you. Dangle your legs, remain silent and rested for a few minutes in that exact position before taking the reading.

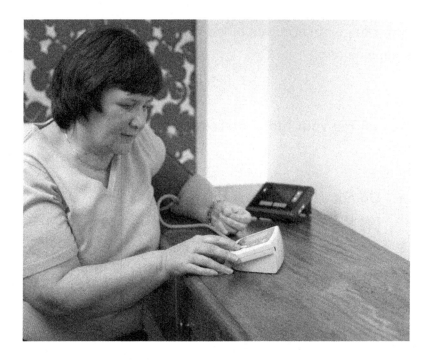

Steps to follow:

1. Wrap the cuff around your upper arm and leave the cuff's lower edge approximately one inch above the bend of your elbow.

2. Put the earpieces of the stethoscope in your ears and place the bell of the stethoscope on your arm over your brachial artery (on your lower arm, just below the edge of the cuff, as in the picture below).

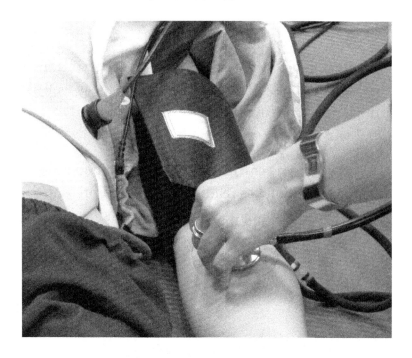

3. **Rapidly inflate the cuff to 180 mm Hg.** At this point you will hear no sound through the stethoscope and no pulse is felt.

4. **Release the air at a rate of around 2 – 3 millimeters per second.** At this point, blood will start to flow through the artery again.

5. **Listen carefully with the stethoscope while looking at the blood pressure monitor.**
   Record the number on the monitor as you hear the first sound in the stethoscope. The first knocking sound, also called the Kortokoff, is the systolic blood pressure (SBP) reading. When the sound stops, record the number on the monitor. This second number is the diastolic blood pressure (DBP) reading.

When taking blood pressure make sure to record the SBP number and the DBP number immediately, as well as which arm was used during the measurement.

Alternatively, you can also buy a digital blood pressure monitor, which makes reading your blood pressure much easier! If you use a digital device, it is still important to have your reading validated and your device calibrated on a regular basis.

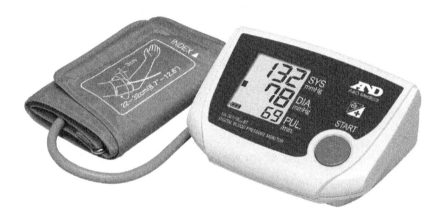

Other things to consider when testing your blood pressure at home is that, when recording your blood pressure, it is also important to record the date and time of the reading. Make sure to check your blood pressure both in the morning and the evening to account for any differences.

Testing your blood pressure at home is a great way to test whether your lifestyle changes are having a positive effect on your blood pressure, and whether or not the prescribed medications are effective. On top of this, it provides you with greater independence as well as constant feedback on your progress – a great source of motivation!

Lastly, it is important to note that blood pressure readings taken at home tend to be lower than normal. Because of this, your blood pressure goal should be 135/85 mm Hg.

5. *Formulating a Successful Treatment Plan*

The first step to creating a successful treatment plan is by setting yourself a clear goal. Your treatment goal will depend on your current blood pressure.

- If you have normal blood pressure (120/80 mm Hg or less), your goal is to keep your blood pressure normal. This can be done by adhering to heart-healthy lifestyle choices.

- If you have prehypertension or high blood pressure (see *subsection 2*), your goal is to lower your blood pressure to the normal range.
    - o If you have prehypertension, it is important to alter your lifestyle habits according to the guidelines provided in *Section 3.*
    - o If you have high blood pressure, apply the same lifestyle modifications. If lifestyle modifications prove to be unsuccessful, consult your physician who may prescribe medications. If medications prove unsuccessful, your doctor may order to have the dosage increased until your blood pressure is under control.

Note that for individuals with kidney disease or diabetes mellitus, the blood pressure goal is 130/80 mm Hg or less.

Therefore, if you are diabetic or have kidney disease and a blood pressure reading of greater than 130/80 mm Hg, then this is considered to be stage 1 hypertension. More information on high blood pressure and diabetes is to be found in *Section 2, subsection 5.*

- If you have a more serious complication associated with high blood pressure, your goal is to control it, prevent it from progressing, and reverse it if possible. Work with your doctor to formulate a plan that could potentially lower your blood pressure or reverse the risk factors. Use the lifestyle modifications outlined in the following sections to supplement your therapy.

You can start taking steps to manage or lower your blood pressure today, regardless of whether your blood pressure is normal, high, or very high. Firstly, however, it is important to differentiate between the habits that have a good effect on your blood pressure and those that have a bad effect on your blood pressure and general health.

Good Habits	Bad Habits
Eating healthily	Salt
Staying physically active	Tobacco
Maintaining a healthy weight	Alcohol
Monitoring your blood pressure	Caffeine

Meditation and Yoga	Stress

The more good habits you adopt, and the more bad habits you eliminate, the greater the effect they are likely to have on your blood pressure. Some people have managed to avoid blood pressure medication altogether by sticking to healthy lifestyle habits. After all, treating high blood pressure is a lifelong focus!

When setting goals, make sure to set long-term goals as well as short-term goals (e.g. your goals for the week and for each day). The following are general guidelines that will help you set achievable and effective goals.

- Always write your goals down.
- Be precise in your daily goals.
- Express your goals in a positive way – use positive statements and positive affirmations. E.g. 'Exercise every day and stay optimistic', rather than 'Don't forget to exercise'.
- Set performance goals, not outcome goals – only set goals over which you have control, e.g. how much to exercise and the types of food to eat and not what your blood pressure reading for that day should be.
- Set priorities – make sure that your daily goals take priority over other less important tasks.
- Set realistic goals.

Tips on how to go about incorporating these lifestyle changes into your daily life can be found in *Section 3* of this guide, along with eating and exercise guidelines and plans. In the next section we will discuss different blood pressure concerns applicable to specific portions of society.

10-Step Treatment Plan to Lower Your Blood Pressure in 4 Weeks!

- **Step 1: Lose 5 pounds** (See *section 3*, subsections 1, 2, 3, 4, Bonus 2 and 3 for strategies and tips on how to loose weight safely and naturally for long-term health.)
- **Step 2: Cut down on salt** (See *section 3, subsection 1* for daily consumption guidelines, as well as tips and tricks on how to cut down on salt.)
- **Step 3: Exercise regularly** (See *Section 3, subsection 4* for exercise guidelines, plans, and motivational tips to help you exercise.)
- **Step 4: Eat the right foods!** (See *Section 3, subsection 2* and 3 for nutritional guidelines and eating plans and Bonus 3 for delicious and nutritious recipes.)
- **Step 5: Try juicing!** (See Bonus 2.)
- **Step 6: Stay away from toxins!** (See *Section 3, subsection 5* for guidelines, techniques, and advice.)
- **Step 7: Eat Potassium!** (See *Section 4, subsection 4* for how potassium can help you lower your blood pressure).

- **Step 8: Manage stress more healthily** (See *Section 4, subsection 1* for methods and tips on how to reduce stress in your life and *subsection 2* for mind-body techniques that can help you manage stress and reduce blood pressure at the same time.)
- **Step 9: Take natural supplements!** (See Bonus 1.)
- **Step 10: Eat dark chocolate!** (See Bonus 1.)

Section 2: Different People, Different Blood Pressure Concerns

In this section we will cover the demographics that are at a particularly high risk for developing high blood pressure, as well as those with different blood pressure management requirements.

1. *Risk Factors for High Blood Pressure*

High blood pressure can affect children, women and men around the world. Despite this, certain factors such as a family history of high blood pressure, race or ethnicity, age, and lifestyle habits appear to have a contributing effect to a person developing high blood pressure. In this section, we will discuss the factors that can increase your risk of developing hypertension.

- **Age:**

The risk of developing high blood pressure is much greater in men aged 55 or above and in women aged 65 or above. This is because high blood pressure naturally rises with age. In the U.S. alone, high blood pressure arises in two-thirds of all individuals aged 65 or above. Special considerations on how to treat high blood pressure in older people will be the focus of the next subsection.

Notably however, there has also been a rise in high blood pressure among children. This recent phenomenon is likely due to the rise in overweight and obese children and adolescents. How to treat high blood pressure in children will be discussed in *subsection 3*.

- **Ethnicity:**

The prevalence of high blood pressure is greater among African American adults when compared to adults with a Caucasian or Hispanic background. Compared to these groups, African American adults have shown to have a higher average high blood pressure, develop high blood pressure at an earlier age, and are less likely to respond to high blood pressure treatment. Because of this, implementation of preventative non-pharmacological treatment, as discussed in *Section 3* of this guide, should be emphasized early.

- **Gender:**

Below the age of 55, men are more likely to develop high blood pressure. From the age of 55 onwards, women are considered to be more likely to develop high blood pressure.

- **Obesity and Overweight:**

Individuals who are obese or overweight are much more likely to develop high blood pressure. Someone who is obese or overweight is defined by having a body weight that is greater than that considered healthy for a certain height.

Obesity and Body Mass Index (BMI)

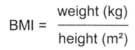

$$BMI = \frac{weight\ (kg)}{height\ (m^2)}$$

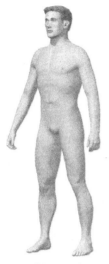 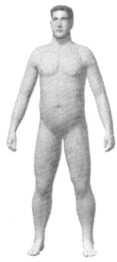 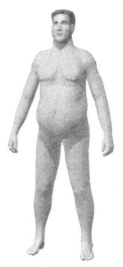

Normal	Overweight	Obese
<25 kg/m²	25 – 29 kg/m²	≥ 30 kg/m²

- **Family History:**

Those with a family history of high blood pressure are at a greater risk of developing prehypertension or hypertension. This genetic link may be due to a sensitivity to sodium and salt, which can run in the family.

- **Bad Lifestyle Habits:**

People with bad lifestyle habits are at a greater risk of developing high blood pressure. Bad lifestyle choices that can raise your risk of high blood pressure include: a lack of physical activity, smoking, drinking too much alcohol or coffee, and eating too much salt or too little potassium.

Lastly, it is important to note that people with high blood pressure, who also have kidney damage, high blood cholesterol or high blood sugar, face even higher risks of developing stroke or heart attacks. If this applies to you, it is thus crucial to also undergo regular check-ups for urine albumin, blood sugar, and blood cholesterol when visiting your doctor.

2. *Treating High Blood Pressure in the Elderly*

More than two-thirds of individuals aged 65 and above experience high blood pressure. On top of this, the elderly are also at greatest risk of a heart or brain attack. The cause of hypertension in most elderly persons is at large unknown. Contributors to the general rise of blood pressure among the elderly may include medications with a blood-pressure-rising effect, diseases and other indeterminable causes.

Systolic High Blood Pressure

In most societies around the world, an individual's systolic pressure rises throughout their life. The same individual will often experience a drop in their diastolic blood pressure from their mid-50s to early-60s. This drop in diastolic blood pressure causes the arteries to stiffen as the individual ages. The ensuing rise in systolic high blood pressure is referred to as 'isolated systolic hypertension' (systolic blood pressure is above 140 mm Hg, whereas the diastolic blood pressure is below 90 mm Hg). In some people, the systolic blood pressure can predict a possible heart or brain attack. When a person aged 65 or above has a systolic blood pressure reading of 140 mm Hg or above, it is important to immediately consult a physician. It is important for that person to commence treatment, either by way of medication and/or lifestyle changes.

Diastolic High Blood Pressure

Diastolic hypertension on the other hand (where the systolic blood pressure is less than 140 mm Hg and the diastolic blood pressure is above 90 mm Hg), is generally not a risk among the elderly population. It is important to note however that if a person's diastolic blood pressure is above 105 mm Hg, that person is nevertheless likely to require treatment and should therefore consult with a doctor.

Blood Pressure Category	Systolic (mm Hg)		Diastolic (mm Hg)
Normal	Less than 120	And	Less than 80
Prehypertension	120 – 139	Or	80 – 90

High Blood Pressure Stage 1	140 – 159	Or	90 – 99
High Blood Pressure Stage 2	160 or higher	Or	100 or higher
Hypertensive Crisis (Emergency Care Needed)	180 or higher	Or	110 or higher

Pseudo High Blood Pressure

Pseudo high blood pressure or pseudo-hypertension is a condition caused by the calcification of arteries. With aging, calcium starts to deposit alongside the artery wall, which can lead to inaccuracies in blood pressure readings. This means that although a person's blood pressure is normal, the meter will register that person's blood pressure as high.

The following are indications that may be suggestive of the possibility of pseudo high blood pressure:

- The person exhibits no other signs of high blood pressure.

- The person exhibits low blood pressure symptoms despite readings indicating high blood pressure.
- Treatment has no or little effects on blood pressure.

If you suspect pseudo high blood pressure, it is advised to consult a doctor who can perform other assessments to get a direct measurement of blood pressure.

Treating elderly patients for high blood pressure, including those who have isolated systolic hypertension, includes following the general guidelines outlined in *Section 3* of this guide. In most cases however, a combination of medications are needed for elderly patients to reach their blood pressure goals.

Postural Low Blood Pressure

Roughly 10% of elderly people will experience postural hypotension (low blood pressure). Postural hypotension is characterized by a sudden fall in blood pressure by as much as 20 mm Hg after standing. The conditions causing blood pressure to drop after standing for long periods, are even more frequent in elderly persons who already have diabetes, adrenal gland failure, or systolic high blood pressure.

Symptoms of postural hypotension include:

- Blurry vision
- Lightheadedness
- Dizziness
- Loss of consciousness

In order to treat or alleviate the effects of postural hypotension, the following approaches may be taken:

- Making sure the person is well hydrated.
- Performing leg exercises – this is to encourage blood backflow and to minimize pooling of blood in the legs.
- Reducing the dose of blood pressure drugs such as alpha and beta blockers.
- Tilting the person's bed to elevate their head.
- Wearing elastic hose – this is because in elderly people, blood tends to remain in the lower part of their body. Wearing elastic hoses discourages pooling of the blood in the legs and helps push blood back to the heart.

Medications That Raise Blood Pressure

Many elderly people suffer from a variety of health related complications which are usually treated with medications. Those that suffer from arthritis for example, are often maintained on NSAIDs (nonsteroidal anti-inflammatory drugs). These drugs provide pain-killing, fever-reducing, and anti-inflammatory effects.

NSAIDs that can be purchased over-the-counter include:

(Brand Name) – Generic Name

- (Advil, Motrin) – **Ibuprofen**
- (Aleve) – **Naproxen Sodium**
- (Ascriptin, Bayer, Ecotrin) – **Aspirin**

NSAIDs that are only available with a doctor's prescription include:

(Brand Name) – Generic Name

- (Anaprox) – **Naproxen Sodium**
- (Celebrex) – **Celecoxib, Sulindac**
- (Daypro) – **Oxaprozin, Salsalate, Diflunisal**
- (Feldene) – **Piroxicam**
- (Indocin) – **Indomethacin, Etodolac**
- (Mobic) – **Meloxicam**
- (Naprosyn) – **Naproxen, Nabumetone, Ketorolac Tromethamine**
- (Vimovo) – **Naproxen/Esomeprazole**
- (Voltaren) – **Diclofenac**

NSAIDs medications specifically include a warning that they cause an increased risk of heart attack, stroke, or stomach bleeding - especially in higher doses. Because of this, an elderly person with high blood pressure who is taking NSAIDs should immediately consult their physician and discontinue the medication if possible. This is because

NSAIDs, particularly when mixed with medication for high blood pressure, block the action of the high-blood-pressure-lowering drug, thereby raising blood pressure.

The following are steps that can be taken to treat high blood pressure in elderly patients:

- Improve nutrition, e.g. by following the DASH diet – the DASH diet may lower blood pressure enough to eliminate the need for medications.
- Reduce salt intake – the lower the salt intake, the lower the blood pressure.
- Reduce alcohol intake.
- Stop smoking.
- Reduce excessive intake of caffeine.
- Increase daily exercise.
- Incorporate mind-body therapies, e.g. meditation and yoga into the daily lifestyle.
- Last resort: taking medications that lower blood pressure.

Positive lifestyle changes that you can adopt will be discussed in greater detail in *Section 3* of this guide. You will also find exercise plans, eating plans, a daily intake guide for caffeine and sodium, and more information on other steps you can take to make your blood pressure goal a reality!

3. *Treating High Blood Pressure in Children*

High blood pressure in children can have different causes, the most common one being obesity and other problems associated with childhood weight. Other risk factors include a family history of high blood pressure, sleep disorders and sleep apnea. High blood pressure in children can result in more serious and long-term health consequences, including stroke, heart and kidney disease.

Normal Blood Pressure in Children

Children begin their lives with a much lower blood pressure. Because of this, it is important to understand the normal progression of blood pressure of your child. This will help you determine when your child's blood pressure is too high.

Newborns / Toddlers Age	Normal Blood Pressure (SBP/DBP in mm Hg)
Newborn	55-75 / 35-45

0-3 months	65-85 / 45-55
3-6 months	70-90 / 50-65
6-12 months	80-100 / 55-65
1-3 years	90-105 / 55-70

The average systolic blood pressure (SBP) of a newborn child ranges from around around 55 mm Hg to 75 mm Hg. Their average diastolic blood pressure (DBP) ranges from 35 mm Hg to 45 mm Hg. However, within a month of birth, the systolic blood pressure can rise to 85 mm Hg and will continue to rise throughout the child's lifetime and into adulthood.

Young Children Age	Normal Blood Pressure (SBP/DBP in mm Hg) Girls	Normal Blood Pressure (SBP/DBP in mm Hg) Boys
Age 3	104-110 / 65-68	104-113 / 63-67
Age 4	105-111 / 67-71	106-115 / 66-71
Age 5	107-113 / 69-73	108-116 / 69-74
Age 6	108-114 / 71-75	109-117 / 72-76

Age 7	110-116 / 73-76	110-119 / 74-78
Age 8	112-118 / 74-78	111-120 / 75-80
Age 9	114-120 / 75-79	113-121 / 76-81
Age 10	116-122 / 77-80	114-123 / 77-82
Age 11	118-124 / 78-83	116-125 / 78-83
Age 12	120-126 / 79-82	119-127 / 79-83

It is important to remember that height can also affect blood pressure. For example, a tall 6-year-old child will exhibit a higher blood pressure reading compared to a short 6-year-old child. Because of this, a tall boy who is healthy will have a maximum blood pressure reading of 125/83 mm Hg at the age of 11, while a short boy of the same age will have a blood pressure reading of 116/78 mm Hg, both of which are considered as being 'within the normal range.'

White Coat Effect or White Coat Hypertension

The white coat effect means that a blood pressure reading in a clinical setting will be higher than the blood pressure reading taken at home. This 'effect' or phenomenon is often caused when a patient is nervous or anxious about having their blood pressure tested by a nurse or doctor (i.e. by a person in a 'white coat'). This makes it difficult to to establish whether a patient actually has high blood pressure. White coat hypertension can cause the systolic blood pressure reading to be around 10 mm Hg higher than usual and elevate the diastolic blood pressure reading by around 5 mm Hg.

The white coat effect is particularly common among children. Because of this, home monitoring of blood pressure, as outlined in *Section 1*, is of utmost importance when dealing with high blood pressure in children.

The Causes of High Blood Pressure

The three main causes of high blood pressure in children and adolescents are typically identified as being hereditary, or as a result of obesity or disease.

Hereditary

High blood pressure – just like height or hair color – can run in the family. Many children with high blood pressure also have adult relatives that suffer from high blood pressure. This indicates a hereditary aspect to hypertension. This link is particularly prevalent among African-American children where there is a higher incidence of high blood pressure.

While one cannot control hereditary risk factors, there are steps that can be taken to live a healthy life, thereby lowering other risks associated with high blood pressure. Healthy lifestyle choices, which will be discussed *Section 3*, have allowed many people with a family history of high blood pressure to avoid high blood pressure altogether.

Disease

When a newborn child has continuous high blood pressure through to 6 years of age, this is usually classified as **secondary high blood pressure**. Secondary high blood pressure is blood pressure resulting from a disease. The most common causes of secondary high blood pressure in this age group (0 – 6 years) is coarctation (congenital narrowing of the aorta), kidney disease, or blockage of one or both arteries to the kidneys.

From the age of 7 onwards, secondary high blood pressure is still common, but **essential blood pressure** starts to appear. Essential blood pressure is blood pressure where the exact cause is unknown. Obesity begins to also have an impact on blood pressure at this age.

- Generally, before the age of 11, most children with high blood pressure (around 90%) will have secondary high blood pressure.
- From the age of 11 onwards, the causes of high blood pressure begin to mirror those of hypertension in adults. Essential blood pressure becomes significantly more common from this age onwards.

Obesity

Obesity is considered the primary cause of high blood pressure in children. It also increases the risk of the child developing other health problems, such as diabetes and heart disease. Obesity is often due to a combination of the following two factors: too much food and too little physical activity.

For children with high blood pressure, lifestyle changes are strongly recommended. Pharmacological intervention should be a method of last resort.

What to Do If Your Child Has High Blood Pressure

When your child has high blood pressure, it is crucial to immediately consult your pediatrician. The doctor should examine the child's medical history, the family history, as well as perform a physical examination to uncover possible causes of high blood pressure.

In most cases, the doctor should be able to pinpoint the cause of high blood pressure after a careful evaluation. In cases where the cause is reversible, e.g. where hypertension is the result of a coarctation of the aorta or an obstruction of an artery leading to the kidney, the doctor might call for surgery. Where the cause is unknown (essential high blood pressure), lifestyle changes can be adopted in order to control high blood pressure. Lifestyle changes, particularly in older children, may be sufficient to reverse the effects of high blood pressure. In some cases, for example where the cause of high blood pressure is secondary, blood pressure medications may be prescribed.

Lastly, it is crucial to have your child's blood pressure checked regularly in order to assess whether blood pressure treatment, whether that is lifestyle changes or the administration of medications, is fruitful.

The following are lifestyle modifications you can adopt to lower your child's blood pressure:

- **Avoid or reduce stress** – if stress is the cause of your child's high blood pressure, or a contributing factor, therapy may be prescribed in order to help your child deal with their concerns and anxieties.
- **Avoid tobacco smoke** – reducing secondary smoke, as will be discussed in *Section 3, subsection 5*.

- **Choose healthy foods** – follow the DASH diet plan by encouraging fresh fruits, vegetables and whole-grain foods. The best way to do this is to make having a balanced diet a family affair. More about a nutritionally balanced diet can be found in *Section 3, subsection 2*. Sample DASH diet plans can be found in *Section 3, subsection 3*.
- **Encourage daily exercise** – it is important for your child to understand that exercising regularly is crucial to health. Encouraging physical activity goes hand in hand with limiting the amount your child spends watching TV or playing video games.
- **Monitoring the weight of your child** – If your child is overweight, it is important to encourage healthy eating and regular exercise to help him or her loose excess weight. It is recommended to consult with your child's doctor or health specialist, who will help your child set weight-loss goals.
- **Eliminate caffeine** – If your child drinks any drinks that contain caffeine, he or she should be encouraged to give up this habit as early as possible.
- **Reduce salt consumption** – Reducing daily salt intake is crucial to lowering blood pressure. We will discuss the effects of salt on blood pressure and how to go about reducing salt in *Section 3, subsection 1*.

Adopting all of the above, or at least a combination of the listed lifestyle modifications, will come a long way in lowering your child's blood pressure. More information on the effect of these lifestyle changes on blood pressure, and how to go about implementing these, are found in *Section 3* of this guide.

4. *High Blood Pressure, Women and Childbearing*

Oral contraceptives increase the risk of blood pressure with duration of use. This is why women who take oral contraceptives should have their blood pressure checked regularly. High blood pressure occurs in approximately 10% of first pregnancies and in around 8% of all pregnancies. It is particularly common in women who have previously taken oral contraceptives for a long period of time. In the U.S. specifically, high blood pressure affects around 6 – 8% of all pregnancies according to the National Heart, Lung, and Blood Institute (NGLBI). Roughly 70% of high blood pressure cases occur in first-time pregnancies.

High blood pressure can be either temporary or permanent and can appear either before or during the pregnancy.

High Blood Pressure Before Pregnancy

Women with high blood pressure or any other related pre-existing condition before or during pregnancy should be monitored carefully because of increased risks to the fetus and the mother herself. If you already have a pre-existing condition (any of those listed below), it is recommended to consult your doctor before becoming pregnant. This is because any pre-existing conditions, particularly those relating to high blood pressure, must be closely monitored and controlled during pregnancy.

If you are taking high blood pressure medication and are intending on become pregnant, it is crucial to first consult your doctor. If you already have high blood pressure, it is also important to keep in mind that a pregnancy can make your high blood pressure even more severe.

If you are pregnant or plan to become pregnant, it is important to consult with your doctor if any of the following applies to you:

- **You have hypertension before becoming pregnant** – In this case, it is important to check with your physician to have your blood pressure checked and also to see whether or not you can stop or reduce your blood pressure medication.
- **You are taking ACE inhibitors or ARBs** – You must immediately notify your doctor if you are taking an ACE inhibitor or an angiotensin receptor blocker and think that you may be pregnant. This is because these medications have shown to be harmful for both the mother and fetus during a pregnancy. If you are planning to become pregnant and are taking any of these medications, it is important to consult your doctor for alternatives.
- **You have kidney disease** – If you suffer from kidney disease, it is important to discuss with your doctor whether pregnancy is advisable. This is because there

is an increased risk of kidney failure with pregnancy. There is however evidence that women with mild kidney disease (stages 1 – 2), normal blood pressure and little to no protein in their urine, can have a healthy pregnancy. For more information on pregnancy and kidney disease, you can visit www.kidney.org.

Whichever of the above conditions you have, it is preferable to consult your physician before becoming pregnant to make sure you understand the risk factors associated with pregnancy in your specific case. By carefully controlling your blood pressure and following the recommendations of your physician, you can increase your chances of having a normal pregnancy and a healthy baby.

High Blood Pressure During Pregnancy

Even if you do not have hypertension or another pre-existing condition, it is nevertheless advisable to visit your doctor before becoming pregnant and to have your blood pressure measured and recorded. This is because there are different factors that can cause high blood pressure during pregnancy. Having your blood pressure measured before pregnancy will allow your doctor to determine whether or not your blood pressure reading is new or whether it has been at that level before your pregnancy. This information is particularly beneficial should you develop high blood pressure during pregnancy.

Preeclampsia

Preeclampsia is a condition in pregnancy which is characterized by high blood pressure and signs of possible damage to other bodily organs such as the kidneys. Preeclampsia can cause fetal complications, harm the placenta, and can cause damage to the kidneys, liver and brain of the mother. The complication usually starts after week 20 of a pregnancy in women and is typically cured with delivery of the baby. Preeclampsia is dangerous for both the mother and the fetus and can cause seizures if left untreated.

The exact cause of preeclampsia is unknown. The risk of developing preeclampsia is greater if any one of the following applies to the patient:

- It is her first baby or it is a baby with a new partner, particularly if the mother is younger than 19 or older than 40.
- She had preeclampsia in a previous pregnancy.
- Her mother had preeclampsia.
- She is carrying twins or triplets (more than one baby).
- She is obese prior to pregnancy.
- She had a pre-existing kidney disease before becoming pregnant.
- She had high blood pressure before becoming pregnant.

- She has diabetes with an associated complication such as kidney disease, nerve disease, or eye disease.

The following are symptoms associated with preeclampsia:

- A large amount of protein in the urine (more than 300 milligrams of protein in urine within a 24-hour period).
- Abdominal pain.
- Blurred vision or changes in vision.
- Excessive or rapid weight gain.
- Headache.
- Swelling.

Preeclampsia can occasionally degenerate into eclampsia, which is a life-threatening condition. Eclampsia is a hypertensive emergency that can give rise to serious health complications such as brain swelling, seizures, kidney failure, blood clotting disorders, pulmonary edema and blindness.

There is currently no proven way to prevent preeclampsia. There is no specific diagnostic test for preeclampsia. High blood pressure, excessive levels of protein in the urine, coupled with any of the above or a combination thereof, however, is usually indicative of preeclampsia.

Preeclampsia and Chronic High Blood Pressure

The treatment of preeclampsia in the presence of high blood pressure must be even more controlled. This is because during a pregnancy, preeclampsia can degenerate into chronic high blood pressure. In the face of this serious complication, termination of the pregnancy may be suggested as a form of curing preeclampsia.

The following are early warning signs of potential preeclampsia in patient with high blood pressure:

- Abnormal liver function.
- Protein in the urine or a sudden increase of protein in the urine.
- A sudden increase in blood pressure (that has previously been controlled).
- A tendency to bleeding (caused by a platelet count of less then 100.000 per cubic millimeter of blood).

The best preventative steps that you can take if you are pregnant are to receive early and regular care and to follow your physician's recommendations. Have your blood pressure checked regularly and manage your blood pressure as much as possible, e.g. by engaging in regular exercise and by limiting salt intake.

Transient (Temporary) High Blood Pressure

High blood pressure during pregnancy is transient or temporary if:

- There is no preeclampsia associated with gestational high blood pressure. No protein is found in the urine and the patient experiences none of the other signs or symptoms associated with preeclampsia.
- The high blood pressure disappears approximately 12 weeks after delivery.

Transient high blood pressure is usually not directly harmful to the mother and fetus and is therefore not treated during pregnancy. It does however tend to reappear in future pregnancies (though it is no particular cause for concern) and is also a warning sign that the mother may, in the future, develop essential high blood pressure. Because of this, mothers who have experienced transient high blood pressure during a past pregnancy should be encouraged to adopt heart-healthy lifestyle modifications. After all, prevention is better than cure!

Lifestyle changes that have a blood-pressure-lowering effect and which can be easily incorporated in one's every day life can be found in *Section 3* of this guide.

5.   *High Blood Pressure and Diabetes Care*

The goal blood pressure reading of a person with diabetes is 130/80 mm Hg or less.

Diabetes is a metabolic disease characterized by elevated blood glucose levels. There are two main types of diabetes:

- **Type 1:** Where your body is unable to produce any insulin. Treatment of type 1 diabetes usually requires daily insulin injections, which is supplemented by living a healthy and balanced lifestyle.

- **Type 2:** Where your body cannot use insulin or does not produce enough insulin. Treatment of type 2 diabetes typically includes leading a healthy and balanced lifestyle alone. At times, insulin injections or tablets may be needed.

Diabetes damages the arteries of the heart and can cause atherosclerosis. Atherosclerosis is a disease characterized by the hardening of the blood vessels, which is caused by the deposit of plaque in the inner walls of the arteries. As seen in the diagram below, this can lead to a narrowing of the arteries, which in turn causes high blood pressure. If left untreated, this can lead to heart failure, blood vessel damage, and stroke.

Normal Artery   Narrowing of Artery

Lipid deposit of
plaque

People with diabetes are therefore at an increased risk of developing high blood pressure. If you have diabetes, it is thus crucial to have your blood pressure regularly monitored and strictly controlled, because high blood pressure can worsen complications associated with diabetes. People diagnosed with diabetes should have their blood pressure measured regularly. This is particularly important because people with diabetes are at an increased risk of developing heart complications at a younger age.

Conversely, having high blood pressure also raises your risk of developing diabetes. Other non-controllable contributing factors that increase your risk include: your age, ethnic background, and a family history of diabetes.

Signs and symptoms of diabetes include:

- Blurred vision or changes in vision.
- Extreme fatigue.
- Frequent need to urinate, particular during the night.
- Increased hunger.
- Increased thirst.
- Weight loss.

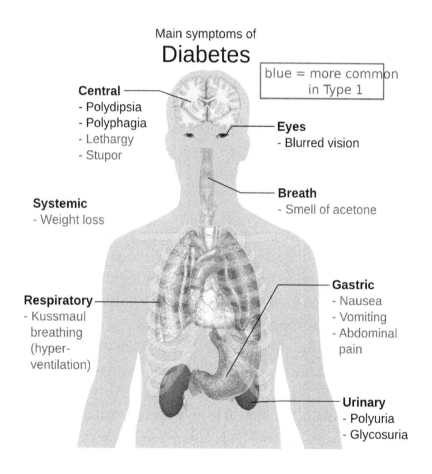

Main symptoms of
Diabetes

blue = more common in Type 1

Central
- Polydipsia
- Polyphagia
- Lethargy
- Stupor

Eyes
- Blurred vision

Breath
- Smell of acetone

Systemic
- Weight loss

Gastric
- Nausea
- Vomiting
- Abdominal pain

Respiratory
- Kussmaul breathing (hyper-ventilation)

Urinary
- Polyuria
- Glycosuria

Managing Diabetes and High Blood Pressure

Blood pressure levels can be lowered through the administration of medications and through the adoption of heart-healthy lifestyle changes. The same lifestyle modifications can be adopted to prevent and control both diabetes and high blood pressure. They include, amongst other things:

- Controlling blood sugar.
- Eating healthy – do the DASH diet!
- Maintaining a healthy body weight.
- Exercising regularly.
- Limiting alcohol consumption.
- Limiting salt intake.
- Quitting smoking.

All of these will be discussed in the following section. However, if you have diabetes and high blood pressure, it is highly recommended to visit your doctor regularly. If you have diabetes and have a blood pressure reading of 140/80 mm Hg or more despite lifestyle modifications, medications are usually advised. There are several available blood pressure medications, but which one you are prescribed will depend on a variety of factors such as your age, your ethnic origin, other medications you take, your medical history, and possible side-effects of the prescribed medication.

Section 3: Treating and Preventing High Blood Pressure

Everyone should have their blood pressure checked on a regular basis. If your blood pressure is high, it is important to seek advice and adopt lifestyle modifications that will help you lower your blood pressure.

For most people, the lifestyle changes outlined in this section will be sufficient to control blood pressure. For others, usually those at stage 2 hypertension, such changes are insufficient and prescription medications are needed to control blood pressure. But even for those receiving pharmacologic treatment, adopting these healthy lifestyle changes is nevertheless critical because they serve to enhance the effectiveness of medications.

At whatever stage you find yourself, there are five key lifestyle changes that you can adopt to prevent or reduce your risk of developing high blood pressure. These will be discussed in turn in this section and broadly include the following: avoiding or reducing salt intake, adopting a healthy diet, avoiding harmful substances, exercising regularly, and managing stress.

1. ***Cutting Down on Salt***

When trying to reduce your blood pressure, salt is your worst enemy. Studies have found that, in most cases, eating less salt leads to lower blood pressure and fewer instances of health complications associated with the heart or brain. Therefore, generally speaking, the lower your salt intake, the lower your blood pressure. This is because excess sodium holds excess fluid in the body, creating an added burden on your heart, thereby increasing blood pressure. Because of this, controlling your salt intake is of utmost importance in lowering your blood pressure and thereby reducing your risk of developing health complications.

In this subsection, we will cover everything you need to know about salt, how to reduce the amount of salt in your diet, which foods are high in salt, which foods are low in salt, as well as tricks and tips to sticking to a low-salt diet!

Sodium: The Truth

It is important to remember that sodium is in many ways our friend as well as our enemy. Sodium is crucial for our body as it maintains the acid and base balance which is necessary for our bodily functions to operate effectively. The normal sodium balance of our body can be maintained by a daily intake of around 3/4 of a teaspoon of salt. Food labels will usually state the amount of sodium content. The dietary guidelines of the American Heart Association recommend a daily intake of 1,500 mg of sodium a day. The average American however, consumes around 3,400 mg of sodium a day.

Contrary to common belief, the biggest contributor to our daily sodium consumption is not table salt – the vast majority (around 75%) of sodium is being consumed through restaurant meals and processed foods.

Sodium Content in Salt

Salt contains around 40% sodium and 60% chloride. The following are the approximate amounts of sodium found in table salt:

- **1/4 teaspoon** salt contains **575 mg sodium**
- **1/2 teaspoon** salt contains **1,150 mg sodium**
- **3/4 teaspoon** salt contains **1,725 mg sodium**
- **1 teaspoon** salt contains **2,300 mg sodium**

The U.S. Food and Drug Administration (FDA) has published the following guidelines for food companies that help you understand the salt content of the products you purchase (accurate as of March 2016: it is important to note that the FDA is currently proposing updates to the Nutrition Facts labels for packaged foods).

- **'Sodium-Free'** means the product contains less than 5 mg of sodium per serving.
- **'Very Low Sodium'** means the product contains 35 mg of sodium or less per serving.
- **'Low Sodium'** means the product contains 140 mg of sodium or less per serving.
- **'Reduced Sodium'** means the product contains at least 25% less sodium than the regular product.
- **'Light in Sodium'** or **'Lightly Salted'** means the product contains at least 50% less sodium than the regular product.
- **'No-Salt-Added'**, **'Without added salt'** or **'Unsalted'** means no salt is added to the product during processing – note however that, unless specifically stated, these products may not be salt or sodium-free.

Making Good Food Choices!

As mentioned earlier, processed food makes up around 75% of our daily sodium intake. Because of this, reducing or cutting processed high-salt foods out of your diet will go a long way in helping you reduce your salt intake and thus manage your blood pressure.

The following is a list of prepared foods that are particularly high in sodium. It is therefore highly recommended to reduce or cut out your intake of such food articles.

Avoid the following food items:

- Anchovies
- Bacon, ham, poultry, sausage, cold cuts and cured meats
- Breads and rolls
- Bouillon cubes
- Canned tuna
- Canned vegetables
- Cheese (natural and processed), particularly cottage cheese
- Condiments
- Cooking sauces, e.g. soy sauce, spaghetti sauce
- Croutons
- Gravy
- Olives
- Pickles
- Pizza
- Prepared meat dishes, e.g. beef stew, chili, and meat loaf
- Prepared pasta dishes, e.g. pasta salad, lasagna, and spaghetti with meat sauce
- Prepared sandwiches, e.g. hamburgers, hot dogs, and submarine sandwiches
- Prepared soups, e.g. canned soup
- Salsa and salad dressings
- Savory snacks, e.g. such as chips, crackers, popcorn, and pretzels
- Tomato and vegetable juice

Tips and Tricks to Reducing Your Salt Intake:

Day-to-day salt-reducing habits:

- Remove the salt from your dining table and hide it in the cupboard!
- Eat fresh, raw vegetables.
- Substitute crisps and other salty snacks with fruits.
- Reduce intake of the following sauces: mustard, ketchup, Worcestershire sauce, and other sauces which are high in salt.
- Reduce intake of salt-cured food.
- Avoid dried fruits that contain salt.
- Avoid processed foods. As a general rule of thumb, the more unprocessed your food and the rawer it is, the lower the salt content.

When buying food:

- Buy fresh foods.
- Check the label! Only purchase products that state the following: 'reduced sodium' or 'no salt added'. As a general rule of thumb, avoid products that contain more than 180 mg of sodium.
- Purchase no-salt or low sodium canned foods.

When cooking:

- When cooking, always use less salt than stated in the recipe.
- Rinse canned foods that contain sodium. This removes the sodium before cooking.
- To flavor your food, substitute salt with herbs, spices, lemon, lime, vinegar, white or red wine.
- Avoid condiments that are high in salt, e.g. soy sauce, teriyaki sauce and anything that contains MSG (monosodium glutamate).
- Avoid salted butter and sauces or dressings that are high in salt.

When eating out:

- When eating out, request your food to be prepared with little salt.
- Request to have sauces, such as salad dressings, served on the side so that you can control the amount you eat.

Potassium helps!

Both potassium and sodium affect blood pressure. Eating foods that are high in potassium, such as bananas, beans, dark leafy greens, potatoes, squash, yogurt, fish, mushrooms and avocadoes, can help you balance out some of the harmful effects that sodium has on your blood pressure.

In summary therefore, in order to promote a lifestyle emphasizing proper nutrition, the following are three general guidelines which you should follow:

- Reduce salt intake to less than 5g of salt per day (i.e. just under a teaspoon).
- Eat at least 5 servings of fruit and vegetables per day.
- Reduce intake of saturated and total fats.

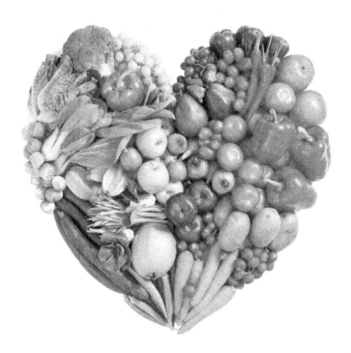

2. *A Slimmer You! – Choosing Foods That Lower High Blood Pressure*

Weight reduction is central to preventing and reducing high blood pressure. Adopting a DASH (Dietary Approaches to Stop Hypertension) eating plan, high in potassium and calcium with sodium restriction, still remains one of the most effective ways in which you can lower your blood pressure. Studies dating back a century have shown that all patients who have adopted a DASH diet have successfully managed to reduce both their systolic and diastolic blood pressure readings.

DASH Theory

DASH emphasizes fruit and vegetable intake. This is because this food category is high in potassium - the higher the potassium, the lower the blood pressure. This correlation is nevertheless dependent on the reduction of salt intake. It is believed that a balanced diet with different nutrients, coupled with reduced salt and increased potassium intake, is responsible for the blood-pressure-lowering effect.

The DASH diet emphasizes good nutrition over calorie counting. A diet that is nutritionally balanced is most important in achieving long-term weight loss success and long-term health benefits.

Among other things, this eating plan has been shown to prevent the following:

- Obesity
- High cholesterol
- Heart disease
- Type 2 Diabetes
- Different forms of cancer

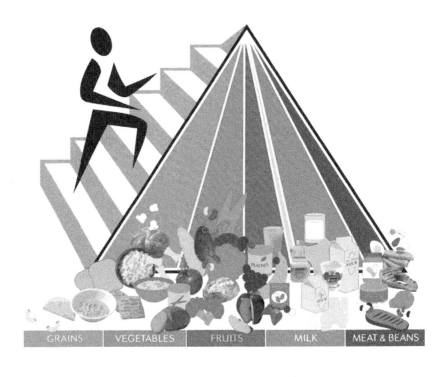

DASH Daily Servings:

1. <u>Vegetables and Fruits: 8 – 10 servings per day</u>

What are good food choices?

- Apples, apple juice
- Apricots
- Artichokes
- Bananas
- Broccoli
- Carrots
- Collards
- Dates
- Grapefruit
- Grapes, grape juice
- Green beans
- Greens
- Kale
- Mangos
- Melons
- Oranges, orange juice
- Peaches
- Peas
- Pineapples
- Prunes
- Spinach

- Squash
- Strawberries
- Sweet potatoes
- Tangerines
- Tomatoes

What is a serving?

- 1 cup of lettuce/other raw leafy vegetables
- ½ cup of other vegetables
- 6 ounces of vegetable juice
- 1 medium fruit
- ½ cup of fresh, frozen, or canned fruit
- ½ cup of dried fruit
- 6 ounces of fruit juice

2. Grains: 7 – 8 servings per day

What are good food choices?

- Cereals that are high in fiber
- English muffins
- Oatmeal
- Pita bread
- Whole wheat bread

What is a serving?

- 1 slice of whole wheat bread
- ½ bagel

- ½ cup of dry cereal
- ½ cup of cooked rice, pasta, or other cereal

3. Dairy (Low-Fat or Fat-Free): 2 – 3 servings per day

What are good food choices?

- Fat-free cheese or part-skim mozzarella
- Fat-free or low-fat yogurt
- Skimmed or 1% fat milk
- Skimmed or low-fat buttermilk

What is a serving?

- 1 cup of milk (1% fat)
- 1 cup of yogurt
- 1 ½ oz. of cheese

4. Fats: 2 – 3 servings per day

What is serving?

- 1 tsp. of olive oil
- 1 tsp. of margarine or mayonnaise
- 1 Tbs. of regular salad dressing
- 2 Tbs. of light salad dressing

5. Seafood, Poultry, or Lean Meat: 0 – 2 servings per day

What are good food choices?

- Lean meat
- Poultry without skin
- Steamed fish/meat (no frying)

What is a serving?

- 3 oz. roasted or broiled seafood, skinless poultry, or lean meat

6. Beans, Nuts & Seeds: 1 serving per day

What are good food choices?

- Almonds, peanuts, mixed nuts
- Kidney beans
- Lentils
- Pinto beans
- Split beans
- Sunflower or sesame seeds
- Tofu

What is a serving?

- 1 cup of cooked beans
- 1/3 cup of nuts
- 2 Tbs. sunflower seeds
- 3 oz. tofu

When selecting your meals, always remember to choose a lower-salt food alternative. On top of the above, you can also incorporate 5 servings of 'sugars' **per week.** Examples of what constitutes a serving include the following:

- 1 cup of low-fat fruit yogurt
- ½ cup of low-fat frozen yogurt
- 1 Tbs. maple syrup, jam, or sugar

Collectively, the above foods will provide you with a nutritionally balanced diet that will not only **boost your metabolism, optimize digestion** and **revitalize your body's fat burning mechanisms,** but also help **reduce cravings** and **control your appetite**!

3. *DASH Diet Eating Plans and Tips*

The DASH diet is based on a 2000-kilocalorie-a-day eating plan that is incredibly easy to incorporate into your daily lifestyle.

Eating Plan 1:

Breakfast	Lunch	Dinner
1 cup corn flakes	2 oz. chicken	3 oz. trout
1 cup 1% milk	½ oz. low-fat cheddar	1 cup rice
1 slice whole wheat bread	1 pita bread	1 cup squash
1 tsp. margarine (even better: 1 tsp. of grass-fed butter)	1 tsp. margarine (even better: 1 tsp. of grass-fed butter)	1 cup spinach or kale
1 tbsp. jam	1 cup raw carrots	1 tbsp. light Italian dressing
1 banana	1 orange	1½ oz. low-fat cheese

**6 oz. orange
juice**

Snacks: 1 medium apple, 1/3 cup of almonds

Eating Plan 2:

Breakfast	Lunch	Dinner
1 cup oatmeal	2 oz. lean beef	3 oz. salmon
1 cup 1% milk	1 tsp. BBQ sauce	1 cup brown rice
1 slice whole wheat bread	1 bread roll	1 cup mixed bean salad
1 tsp. margarine (even better: 1 tsp. of grass-fed butter)	1 ½ oz. low-fat cheddar	1 tbsp. low-fat dressing
1 mango	1 cup of sweet potatoes	1 cup spinach
6 oz. prune	1 cup	1½ oz.

juice	lettuce salad	cornbread muffin
	1 tbsp. low-fat salad dressing	

Snacks: 1 orange, 1 oz. dried fruit, 2 tbsp. sunflower seeds

Don't know what to cook? Don't worry, DASH diet recipes and food ideas can be found in the bonus section at the end of this guide!

Tips that will make sticking to the *DASH Diet* easier:

1. Do not turn your diet around one day to another. It is important to gradually get used to your new heart-healthy eating plan. Slowly increase your intake of fruits and vegetables day by day.
2. Increase your vegetable and fruit intake by having two servings with each meal and two servings during the day for a snack.
3. Use lactose-free milk or take lactase pills if you are lactose intolerant.
4. Check your food labels! Always select the food product with the lowest amount of salt, cholesterol and saturated fats.
5. Replace animal fats with vegetable fats.
6. Avoid drinking alcohol, soda or other sugary drinks.
7. Don't know what to have for dessert? Choose fruits!
8. Base your meals around vegetables, beans and grains (instead of meat, fish, or poultry).

4. *A Fitter You! – Exercises that Lower High Blood Pressure*

Maintaining a normal and healthy weight is crucial in controlling blood pressure. Studies monitoring the effects of weight loss on blood pressure have shown that for every 5 kg of excess weight lost, systolic blood pressure decreases by 2 – 10 points.

Your heart is a muscle and like all the other muscles in your body, it must be exercised to become stronger and more efficient. Of course, besides lowering blood pressure, there are also many other health benefits that flow from regular physical activity.

Sticking to a regular exercise program:

- Boosts your sex drive.
- Controls your weight.
- Improves mental health and mood.
- Improves your memory.
- Increases energy levels.
- Lowers your blood sugar (which also reduces your risk for type 2 diabetes).
- Lowers your risk of some cancers (such as breast cancer and large intestinal cancer).
- Strengthens your bones and muscles.

The above list, of course, is not exhaustive. But hopefully it provides sufficient reason for you to leave your sedentary lifestyle behind you and become an active and happier person!

IMPORTANT: Do note however that if you have not exercised for a couple of years, it is important to consult your doctor before jumping straight into an exercise routine. Make sure to clear any new exercise programs with your physician. If you are aged 40 or above, you should first undergo a physical examination to determine your current physical condition. This will ultimately determine the type of exercise plan that fits your current fitness level, and will help you avoid any potential injuries.

Before starting your exercise program, it is important to keep the following in mind:

- Start slowly and progress gradually. Getting to your goal takes time and the key to healthy exercising is persistence and routine.
- Exercising **daily** (rather than three or four times a week) has a much greater effect on your blood pressure. This is because people with high blood pressure will experience a drop in blood pressure for around 7 – 8 hours after exercising. In the long-term,

regular exercise will have a huge and long-lasting effect on your blood pressure and health.

- Aerobic exercises (e.g. walking, running, swimming, cycling, tennis, etc.) have a much greater effect on your blood pressure compared to anaerobic exercise (e.g. lifting heavy weights). Regular aerobic exercise can with time lower your blood pressure by 10 mm and help you get off blood pressure medications.
- Engaging in a program that contains aerobic, anaerobic and stretching exercises is without doubt the best form of exercise - not only will this lower your blood pressure, but also strengthen your muscles.

You might be unsure about how to gradually increase your exercise goals. The following is a sample 8-week exercise program to help you kick-start your fitness routine with plenty of motivation!

8 Week Exercise Program for Beginners

Week 1	• 2 days of brisk walking or other aerobic exercises (20 minutes each) • 1 weight training session
Week 2	• 3 days of brisk walking or other aerobic exercises (20 – 30 minutes each) • 2 weight training sessions

Week 3	• 4 days of brisk walking or other aerobic exercises (30 minutes each) • 2 weight training sessions
Week 4	• 4 days of brisk walking or other aerobic exercises (30 minutes each) • 3 weight training sessions
Week 5	• 5 days of brisk walking or other aerobic exercises (30 minutes each) • 3 weight training sessions
Week 6	• 5 days of brisk walking or other aerobic exercises (30 – 45 minutes each) • 3 weight training sessions
Week 7	• 6 days of brisk walking or other aerobic exercises (30 – 45 minutes each) • 3 weight training sessions
Week 8	• 5 days of brisk walking or other aerobic exercises (45 – 60 minutes each) • 3 weight training sessions

Aerobic exercises (cardiovascular exercises): help lower your blood pressure and make your heart stronger.

Anaerobic exercises (strength training): good for your bones and joints and helps you build strong muscles that burn more calories throughout the course of the day.

Stretching exercises: help prevent injury and make you more flexible.

The following is an example exercise schedule which combines a healthy amount of aerobic and anaerobic exercises with a focus on aerobic:

Sunday	Monday	Tuesday	Wednesday	Thursday	Friday	Saturday
Walking	Biking	Running for 20 & Strength Training (weights) for 10	Swimming	Strength Training (resistance)	Hiking	Tennis

Min. 30 minutes per day.
Always remember to warm up and stretch for at least 5 minutes before starting any vigorous physical activity!

The following is a 30-minute home strength training work-out of moderate intensity. All you need is a yoga mat and motivation. Gradually add weights to increase intensity.

Warmup: 5 minute stretching or cardio of choice

50 seconds mountain climbers

10 second rest

50 seconds push-ups or plank

10 second rest

50 seconds bicycle crunches

10 second rest

50 seconds jumping jacks or burpees

10 second rest

50 seconds squats or wall sit

10 second rest

REPEAT 5 Times

If running is your goal, the following is a sample 8-week running program for complete beginners. It is important to keep in mind that speed should not be the goal - steady progression is the key. Walk for at least 3 minutes before and after running, listen to your body throughout and most importantly, have fun and stay optimistic!

8 Week Running Program for Beginners

Month 1

Week 1	**Sunday:** Rest day
	Monday: Run 2 minutes, Walk 2 minutes (5 Repeats)
	Tuesday: 25 minutes of brisk walking
	Wednesday: Run 2 minutes, Walk 2 minutes (5 repeats)
	Thursday: 25 minutes of brisk walking
	Friday: 30 minutes of strength training
	Saturday: Rest day

Week 2   **Sunday:** Rest day

Monday: Run 3 minutes, Walk 2 minutes (5 repeats)

Tuesday: 30 minutes of brisk walking

Wednesday: Run 3 minutes, Walk 3 minutes (5 repeats)

Thursday: 30 minutes of brisk walking

Friday: 30 minutes of strength training

Saturday: 20 minutes of stretching/yoga

Week 3   **Sunday:** Rest day

Monday: Run 4 minutes, Walk 2 minutes (5 repeats)

Tuesday: 30 minutes of brisk walking

Wednesday: Run 4 minutes, Walk 3 minutes (5 repeats)

Thursday: 30 minutes of brisk walking

Friday: 30 – 45 minutes of strength training

Saturday: 30 minutes of stretching/yoga

Week 4   **Sunday:** Rest day

Monday: Run 5 minutes, Walk 1 minutes (5 repeats)

Tuesday: 30 minutes of brisk walking

Wednesday: Run 10 minutes, Walk 5 minutes (2 repeats)

Thursday: 30 minutes of brisk walking

Friday: 30 – 45 minutes of strength training

Saturday: 30 minutes of stretching/yoga

From Walker to Runner

Month 2

Week 5   **Sunday:** Rest day

Monday: Run 8 minutes, Walk 2 minutes (3 repeats)

Tuesday: 30 minutes of brisk walking

Wednesday: Run 12 minutes, Walk 3 minutes (2 repeats)

Thursday: 30 minutes of brisk walking

Friday: 30 – 45 minutes of strength training

Saturday: 30 minutes of stretching/yoga

Week 6	**Sunday:** Rest day

Monday: Run 15 minutes, Walk 2 minutes (2 repeats)

Tuesday: 30 minutes of brisk walking

Wednesday: Run 15 minutes, Walk 2 minutes (2 repeats)

Thursday: 30 minutes of brisk walking

Friday: 30 – 60 minutes of strength training

Saturday: 30 – 60 minutes of stretching/yoga

Week 7	**Sunday:** 30 – 60 minutes of stretching / yoga

Monday: Run 15 minutes, Walk 1 minutes (2 repeats)

Tuesday: 30 minutes of brisk walking

Wednesday: Run 10 min., Walk 2 min., Run 20 min.

Thursday: 30 – 60 minutes of strength training

Friday: Run 10 min., Walk 2 min., Run 20 min.

Saturday: 30 minutes of brisk walking

Week 8   **Sunday:** 30 – 60 minutes of stretching / yoga

Monday: Run 26 minutes, Walk 4 minutes (1 time)

Tuesday: 30 minutes of brisk walking

Wednesday: Run 28 minutes, Walk 2 minutes (1 time)

Thursday: 30 – 60 minutes of strength training

Friday: Run 30 minutes (1 time)

Saturday: 30 minutes of brisk walking

Walking Your Way to a Healthy Heart!

Don't worry if you can't run, don't like running or prefer starting with moderate exercises. A study by the Life Sciences Division, conducted at the Lawrence Berkeley Natural Laboratory in Berkley, California, has shown that moderate walking lowers your risk of developing high blood pressure, high cholesterol, and diabetes mellitus just as much as running. The same energy used for moderate and vigorous exercise produces similar reductions. Therefore, the more you walk or run every week, the greater the health benefits.

These findings are consistent with the recommendations of the American Heart Association, which recommends at least 30 minutes of exercise per day. So, in order to reap the health benefits of exercise, you should engage in at least 150 minutes of moderate activity or 75 minutes of vigorous exercise per week.

Remember that 30 minutes of physical activity per day should be the minimum. In the long-term, it will make a huge difference in improving your blood pressure and general health. An alternative to 30-minutes of brisk walking is walking 10,000 steps a day. Use a pedometer and keep track of your daily step count. You should aim to increase your step count by 500 every day until you reach 10,000!

Tips for Staying Motivated and Active!

- Exercise at the same time every day so that exercise becomes part of your regular routine.
- Always wear comfortable clothes when exercising.
- Record your blood pressure before and after exercising. This allows you to really see and

understand the drastic benefits of exercise on lowering your blood pressure.
- Set realistic goals – start small and think big!
- Make it fun: switch up exercises every day (alternate between running, walking, strength training, stretching and different cardiovascular exercises).
- Exercise with a friend or join a club.

In summary therefore, it is important to remember that any type of physical activity, even low-intensity exercises such as walking, can lower your blood pressure in the long-term. Always remember to engage in at least 30 minutes of regular physical activity a day. The health benefits of exercise are substantial and without doubt worth the effort!

5. **_The Triple Cure: Say No to Alcohol, Caffeine, and_**
   Tobacco

By saying no to alcohol, caffeine and tobacco, you will:

- Improve your work performance.
- Improve your sex life.
- Increase your life expectancy.
- Lower your blood pressure.

Most people will find it hard to cut these out permanently. Cutting down on one or hopefully all of these however will go a long way in improving your blood pressure and your overall health.

Please note that alcohol, caffeine, and tobacco are covered in this section only in relation to their effects on high blood pressure. For those wishing to either gain a complete understanding as to the effects and consequences of these stimulants on health, or for those wishing to quit drinking or smoking, information and links to resources that provide comprehensive information, advice, help and guidelines are provided at the end of each subsection.

Alcohol and High Blood Pressure

Alcohol raises blood pressure. Blood pressure falls back to normal once the drinking stops. While drinking in moderation will not have long-term adverse effects on your blood pressure, individuals who drink excessively over long periods of time will experience a persistent rise in their blood pressure.

Besides raising blood pressure, alcohol abuse raises the risk of brain attacks and other health complications, such as heart disease, depression, degeneration of the brain, and an increased risk of cancer. Because of this, alcohol consumption should be moderated.

How Much Is Too Much?

The following is considered to be 'moderate' and reducing alcohol consumption to these levels has shown to reduce blood pressure by 2 – 4 mm Hg (note that this is time-dependent and for some individuals, reducing consumption of these substances could have an even greater effect on lowering blood pressure):

- **Men:** 2 drinks per day for most men
- **Women:** 1 drink per day for most women

What is a drink? A drink classed as 1 oz. or 30 mL ethanol:

- 24 oz. beer
- 10 oz. wine
- 3 oz. whiskey (40% alcohol)

If you are suffering from alcoholism and wish to recover, please refer to the following resources:

- Alcoholics Anonymous (AA): www.aa.org.
- National Council on Alcoholism and Drug Dependence (NCADD): www.ncadd.org.

Tobacco and High Blood Pressure

Smoking is widely known to irritate the lungs, thereby compromising your lung's functional abilities. What is less known however, is that smoking also has an adverse effect on your blood pressure. The nicotine in tobacco elevates blood pressure by constricting your blood vessels. Because of this, the more you smoke, the higher your chances of having high blood pressure.

Studies have shown a direct correlation between the use of tobacco products and hypertension. They have also shown that once a person quits smoking, their blood pressure also falls. It is nevertheless important to bear in mind that blood pressure elevation is just one of many adverse health consequences caused by smoking.

If You Are a Smoker: Quit Smoking

If you are a smoker and have high blood pressure, quitting smoking will certainly come a long way in lowering your blood pressure. Once you quit smoking, your heart and lungs will usually start to function more normally again within 12 hours, thereby lowering your blood pressure.

The following are a few effective methods that can help you quit:

- Nicotine-replacement therapy, e.g. using nicotine gum, nicotine lozenge and nicotine patches.
- Taking medication that facilitate smoking-cessation, such as *Chantix* or *Zyban,* which help reduce withdrawal symptoms.

For more information on how to quit smoking, please refer to the following resources. These organizations and their websites provide information on the impact of smoking on health, along with comprehensive tips and guidelines on quitting smoking and avoiding secondhand smoke:

- Agency for Healthcare Research and Quality (HRQ): www.ahrq.gov.
- American Cancer Society: www.cancer.org.

- National Cancer Institute (NCI): www.cancer.gov.

The following provide both guidelines on quitting smoking, as well as information on clinics and healthcare sites that provide smoking cessation programs:

- American Heart Association: www.heart.org.
- American Lung Association: www.lungusa.org.

If You Are a Non-Smoker: Avoid Side-Stream Tobacco

Side-stream tobacco, or secondhand smoke, is smoke that is inhaled from another person's cigarette. Side-stream tobacco can be just as harmful for your health and should therefore be avoided whenever possible.

In a similar vein, it has likewise been argued that secondhand smoke can be even more harmful than firsthand smoke because it is 'unfiltered', and therefore contains most of the 'bad stuff', including nicotine.

The following are steps you can take to avoid or reduce side-stream tobacco:

- Do not allow anyone to smoke inside your home or car.
- If exposure to smoke cannot be avoided, try and improve ventilation, e.g. through opening windows.

Caffeine and High Blood Pressure

Although the case against caffeine is nowhere as strong as
that against alcohol or tobacco, caffeine has also shown to
temporarily increase blood pressure. Moderate coffee
drinking will not usually cause any long-term damage. A
habit to overdrink on heavily caffeinated coffee on the other
hand, can cause persistent high blood pressure. Studies have
found a blood pressure increase of 5 mm Hg in some people
who drink 4 – 5 of high-caffeinated cups of coffee a day.
Besides spikes in blood pressure, excessive consumption of
caffeine (over 300 mg of caffeine on a daily basis over an
extended period of time) can have potential medical
consequences, including heartburn, insomnia, increased risk
of heart disease, birth complications, and osteoporosis
(thinning of the bones).

Again, people who already have high blood pressure are
more prone to experiencing an increase in blood pressure
due to excess caffeine intake. But even if you do not have
high blood pressure, caffeine has been seen to cause short
but drastic increases in blood pressure. The effects of
caffeine on blood pressure are still widely debated, with
some researchers believing that caffeine blocks a hormone

that helps arteries widen.

Coffee and tea however are not the only source of caffeine: a bottle of cola (16 oz.) contains around 40 mg of caffeine, a 100-gram bar of milk chocolate has around 20 mg of caffeine, and 100 grams of dark chocolate contains 43 mg of caffeine.

How Much Is Too Much?

The general recommendation is not to exceed an intake of 300 mg of caffeine per day. A standard coffee (5 oz.) will contain around 100 mg of caffeine. However, if you already have high blood pressure it is recommended to limit your daily caffeine intake to around 200 mg. It is important to keep in mind that caffeine content of beverages varies by brand and type of drink.

Coffee Type	Size	Caffeine Content
Brewed	8 oz. (237 mL)	95 – 200 mg
Brewed (decaffeinated)	8 oz. (237 mL)	2 – 12 mg

Specialty drink, e.g. latte or mocha	8 oz. (237 mL)	63 – 175 mg
Brewed, single-serve cups	8 oz. (237 mL)	75 – 150 mg
Brewed, single-serve cups (decaffeinated)	8 oz. (237 mL)	2 – 4 mg
Espresso	1 oz. (30 mL)	47 – 75 mg
Espresso (decaffeinated)	1 oz. (30 mL)	0 – 15 mg
Instant	8 oz. (237 mL)	27 – 173 mg
Instant (decaffeinated)	8 oz. (237 mL)	2 – 12 mg

On top of this, it is advised to avoid consuming caffeine before exercising as exercise naturally increases your blood pressure. If you plan to cut down on your caffeine intake, it is also advised to do so gradually over a week or two in order to avoid withdrawal headaches.

For more information on the caffeine content of various food items and medications, the Center for Science in the Public Interest offers and extensive list which can be found on their website (www.cspinet.org) under the following link: www.cspinet.org/new/cafchart.htm.

In summary, to live a healthy lifestyle and control your blood pressure:

- Avoid excessive drinking of alcohol, for example by limiting intake to no more than one regular drink a day.
- Quit smoking and exposure to tobacco products.
- Reduce your caffeine intake to two standard cups or one strong cup of coffee a day.

Treating and Preventing High Blood Pressure: Summary

The benefits of lifestyle modifications on your blood pressure cannot be emphasized enough. Positive lifestyle changes do not only help lower blood pressure, they also enhance the efficiency of antihypertensive medication and decrease the risk of cardiovascular disease. Sticking to the DASH diet plan for example, can be as effective as drug therapy. Lastly, it is important to remember that the lifestyle modifications listed in this section are cumulative. That means that a combination of two, or ideally multiple modifications, can achieve even better long-lasting results.

Section 4: Enhancing Your Hypertension Treatment

The blood-pressure-lowering strategies outlined here are designed to supplement and enhance your existing blood pressure therapy, which should focus on the methods and modifications discussed in the previous section.

1. *__Managing Stress Healthily__*

Mental health has long been neglected by the medical community. A mental injury however can be as harmful as a physical injury. We often underestimate the impact our emotional health has on our cardiovascular health.

Stressful situations and intense stress has actually shown to cause a spike in our blood pressure. Although stress is not a confirmed contributor or risk fact for high blood pressure, stress certainly has an effect on our bodies and overall health. When we experience stress, our body releases stress hormones into our blood system. These stress hormones cause our heart to beat faster, thereby constricting blood vessels and raising our blood pressure temporarily. Over time, repeated instances of short-term stress could increase our risk of eventually developing high blood pressure.

Currently however, there is no proof that stress or negative emotions alone can cause long-term high blood pressure. Rather, it has been suggested that stress is sometimes directly linked to bad blood-pressure-raising habits, including poor sleeping habits, drinking too much alcohol, and overeating.

Whether it is for health reasons or for your own personal wellbeing, learning to cope with stress and stressful situations is definitely a lifestyle habit worth acquiring. As with any other endeavor however, learning to manage stress healthily takes practice and time.

The following are some ways in which you can reduce and control your relationship with stress:

- **Exercise regularly:** Exercise releases endorphins and regular exercise can reduce your stress levels.

- **Know what brings you pleasure and nurture this:** Whether this is going on a long relaxing walk, reading a book or nurturing encouraging relationships.

- **Practice gratitude**: Changing your outlook by focusing on the positive will transform the way you look at life's fallbacks.

- **Relax and take time to care for yourself**: Be conscientious to take time every day to focus on yourself and the present moment.

- **Saying no:** It is important to pinpoint your priorities and to understand your own limitations.

- **Sometimes you cannot control what happens to you, but you can control how you feel about it:** Understand what is out of your control and learn to accept that there are things that you cannot change. The only thing you can control are your emotions, not to be affected by that which has happened but to focus on yourself.

- **Time management:** Allow yourself enough time to get things done.

- **Understand what causes your stress:** Whether this is a relationship with a friend or rush-time traffic. If you can avoid these stress triggers, make sure that you do.

In addition to these methods, there are alternative mind-body techniques and practices that can be employed for effective stress management. If practiced regularly and over a sustained period of time, these can also help control your blood pressure.

2. *Alternative Mind-Body Techniques and Practices to Reduce High Blood Pressure*

"The natural healing force within each one of us is the greatest force in getting well."

- *Hippocrates (c. 460 BC – c. 375 BC)*

Alternative mind-body practices are relaxation techniques that can be used to reduce stress and to lower blood pressure. The mind-body methods discussed in this section can also help treat chronic pain, asthma, anxiety, diabetes, depression, headaches, incontinence, insomnia and panic disorders. It is important to note that the exact effects of mind-body techniques on blood pressure still remain unclear.

All of the methods outlined in this section also help with stress management. Note also that stress can also be reduced using appropriate physical exercise as well as through positive social contact. Importantly, the mind-body therapies outlined here should not replace reducing salt, loosing weight, stopping smoking, or your blood pressure medication. Instead, they should be used as a way of enhancing existing blood-pressure-lowering treatments.

Mind-body methods discussed in this section include the following: meditation, hypnotherapy (hypnosis) and biofeedback.

Meditation

Meditation is the practice of sitting still and connecting with the present moment through focusing on one's breath. Meditation has shown to have numerous health benefits and is commonly employed to relieve stress, anxiety, depression, insomnia, and the symptoms of cancer or cardiovascular disorders. It is used to induce positive emotions and mental calmness.

Adopting a regular meditation practice can help you maintain a focused and calm mind. Meditation can affect your blood pressure because when you are in a relaxed and calm state, your body produces nitric oxide. Nitric oxide helps your blood vessels open up, thereby reducing your blood pressure.

Meditation can be practiced from the comfort of your own home. To ease you into meditation, there is a great variety of different apps, podcasts and online videos available for guided meditation. Across the country, there are also many different meditation centers that offer drop-in meditation classes that only ask for a small donation.

Hypnotherapy

Hypnotherapy or hypnosis is a practice whereby a person is guided into a state of heightened attention and relaxation. Hypnotherapy can be used to alleviate the psychological factors associated with headaches, anxiety and phobias, amongst other things. In some instances, hypnotherapy has helped people quit smoking and lose weight, both of which have a positive effect on blood pressure.

Biofeedback

Biofeedback is a technique that is used by trained people to control body functions that normally occur involuntary, such as blood pressure and heart rate. There are many different biofeedback methods your therapist may use. Biofeedback can be effective for a few conditions but it is primarily used to treat migraines, headaches and chronic pain.

For more information, including a directory of licensed hypnotherapists, hypnosis practitioners or biofeedback specialists near you, you can contact the Association for Applied Psychophysiology and Biofeedback (AABP): www.aapb.org.

Mind-body techniques can be used to supplement and enhance your current blood pressure therapy and can be very effective when combined with the proven blood-pressure-lowering lifestyle changes discussed in *section 3*. However, bear in mind that whilst mind-body techniques are generally safe, they do have their own risks and possible side effects. Because of this, it is advised to consult your health care provider should you have any concerns.

3. _Avoiding Drugs and Supplements That Can Raise Blood Pressure_

Just as there are drugs that have blood-pressure-lowering effects, there are also drugs that can contribute to high blood pressure.

Pain Medications

As mentioned previously, NSAIDs, both prescription and over-the-counter versions, can elevate blood pressure by making your body retain fluid, thereby decreasing the function of your kidneys.

Common used NSAIDs that raise blood pressure include:

- Ibuprofen (e.g. Advil) and
- Naproxen (Anaprox, Aleve).

Other pain medications which can cause blood pressure to rise include:

- Indomethacin (e.g. Indocin) and
- Piroxicam (Feldene).

Besides NSAIDs, there are also many other drugs and supplements which can raise blood pressure, which will be covered in this section.

Cough Medications (Decongestants)

Cough medications often contain NSAIDs and many also contain decongestants. Decongestants can make your blood pressure and heart rate rise. If you are on blood pressure medication, decongestants can prevent these from working properly.

Examples of decongestants include:

- Phenylephrine (Neo-Synephrine).
- Pseudoephedrine (Sudafed).

If you have a cold or cough and have high blood pressure, or are at risk of developing high blood pressure, consult your physician regarding alternative cough medications such as nasal sprays or antihistamines.

Headache Medications

Some medications used to treat headaches or migraines can also raise blood pressure. If you have high blood pressure, it is advised to consult your doctor before taking any drugs to treat your headache or migraine.

Antidepressants

Antidepressants contain chemicals that can cause a spike in your blood pressure. Antidepressants that have blood-pressure-raising effects include:

- Fluoxetine (e.g. Prozac and Sarafem),
- Monoamine oxidase inhibitors.
- Tricyclic antidepressants.
- Venlafaxine (Effexor XR).

If you are taking antidepressants, it is advised to have your blood pressure checked regularly. If you have high blood pressure and are taking antidepressants, it is strongly advised to talk to your doctor to discuss alternative prescriptions.

Birth control

As mentioned previously, birth control pills may increase your blood pressure. If you are currently taking birth control pills or are pregnant and used to take birth control pills over a long period of time, it is advised you to have your blood pressure checked regularly.

Immunosuppressants

Immunosuppressants can affect your kidney function and some can also cause your blood pressure to rise. Examples of immunosuppressants that can raise your blood pressure include:

- Cyclosporine (Neoral, Sandimmune) and
- Tacrolimus (Prograf).

If you are taking any immunosuppressants, it is recommended to have your blood pressure measured on a regular basis, and to consult with your doctor should you have high blood pressure.

Herbal supplements

It is always important to inform your doctor if you are taking any herbal supplements. It is always advised to check with your doctor before taking any herbal supplements. This is particularly important if you have high blood pressure - be aware that some supplements can raise your blood pressure or interfere with your blood pressure medication.

Herbal supplements that can affect your blood pressure include the following:

- Arnica
- Bitter Orange
- Ephedra
- Ginkgo
- Ginseng
- Guarana
- Licorice
- Senna
- St. John's Wort

4. *Fighting Salt with Potassium*

As covered in the previous section, cutting back on salt will come a long way in helping you lower your blood pressure. Just as sodium in salt-sensitive individuals causes blood pressure to rise, there are other electrolytes or minerals that have an effect on our blood pressure. Increasing intake of potassium, calcium and magnesium have all shown to be inversely associated with blood pressure.

Studies experimenting with potassium restrictions have shown that too little potassium has the same effect on blood pressure as too much salt. Because of this, a diet that includes a variety of natural sources of potassium is crucial to controlling blood pressure. Potassium also helps balance out the negative effects of sodium on blood pressure.

The recommended daily intake of potassium to help you lower your blood pressure is roughly **4.7 grams (4,700 milligrams).**

Food labels will usually list how much potassium a product contains. Yet, the best source of potassium is derived from natural and raw products. The following list is designed to give you a general indication of some common food items and their respective potassium contents.

FOOD ITEM (How much?) = POTASSIUM CONTENT (in mg)

- Acorn squash (1 cup) = 900
- Avocado (1/2 medium avocado) = 680
- Banana (1 medium banana) = 451
- Cantaloupe (1 cup) = 450
- Cooked spinach (1 cup) = 839
- Dates (10 whole) = 541
- Dried apricots (10 halves) = 482
- Dried figs (5 whole) = 666
- Honeydew melon (1/4 melon) = 940
- Mango (1 medium mango) = 323
- Orange (1 medium orange) = 250
- Orange juice (1 cup) = 450
- Potato (baked) (1 medium potato) = 844
- Prunes (10 medium prunes) = 626
- Raisins (1/2 cup) = 375
- Strawberries (1 cup) = 247
- Sweet potato (1 cup) = 950
- Tomato puree (1/2 cup) = 525
- Winter squash (1/2 cup) = 445

Generally speaking, you should try to at least incorporate 3.5 grams of potassium in your diet every day, but ideally 4.7 grams. There are many additional benefits that flow from having a diet rich in potassium. Not only does potassium help lower your blood pressure, it also helps stabilize your heartbeat and prevent kidney stones.

In order to ensure that you consume a healthy amount of potassium, try to eat at least 5 portions of fruit and vegetables every day. This will give you a good source of potassium (as opposed to the potassium derived from potassium supplement tablets).

IMPORTANT: If you have kidney disease, increasing your intake of potassium can be harmful. In this case, it is advised to consult your physician or health specialist to devise an eating plan that suits your needs.

5. *Balancing Your Electrolytes: Calcium and Magnesium*

Potassium, compared to calcium and magnesium, has shown to have the greatest, although still relatively modest, blood-pressure-lowering effect in people with an unbalanced diet and electrolyte imbalances. Despite this, calcium and magnesium are essential minerals needed by our body, which are particularly important for our cardiovascular health.

Calcium helps our body maintain and build strong bones. It also helps maintain the proper functioning of our muscles, nerves and heart rhythm.

Magnesium supports our energy metabolism and is essential in maintaining muscle activity, body temperature, and proper nerve function. Some studies have also suggested that calcium and magnesium both have health benefits beyond the above listed, such as protecting against high blood pressure, diabetes and cancer.

How Much Calcium?

Age group	Recommended daily intake of calcium	Maximum daily intake (not to be overstepped)
Infants 0 – 6 months	200 mg	1000 mg
Infants 7 – 12 months	260 mg	1500 mg
Children 1 – 3 years	700 mg	2500 mg
Children 4 – 8 years	1000 mg	2500 mg
Children 9 – 18 years	1300 mg	3000 mg
19 – 50 years Men and Women	1000 mg	2500 mg
51 – 70 years Women	1200 mg	2000 mg
Men	1000 mg	2000 mg

71 years and older Men and Women	1200 mg	2000 mg
Pregnant and Breastfeeding Women 14 – 18 years 19 – 50 years	1300 mg 1000 mg	3000 mg 2500 mg

By eating a variety of the following foods, such as dairy products, dark leafy vegetables and fish, you can ensure that you receive the recommended amount of calcium. The following list is designed to give you a general indication of some healthy food items and their respective calcium contents.

FOOD ITEM (How much?) = CALCIUM CONTENT (in mg)

- Anchovies, canned (75 g) = 174
- Beans, canned or cooked (2/3 cup, 175 ml) = 93 – 141
- Cheese, e.g. goat, low-fat cheddar or mozzarella (50 g) = 395 – 506
- Cooked or frozen kale (1/2 cup) = 95
- Cooked spinach (1/2 cup) = 129
- Cottage cheese (1 cup) = 146 – 217
- Orange juice (1/2 cup, 125 ml) = 155

- Salmon, canned with bones (75 g) = 179 – 208
- Yogurt (3/4 cup, 175 g) = 292 – 332

How Much Magnesium?

Age	Recommended daily intake of magnesium
Infants 0 – 6 months	30 mg
Infants 7 – 12 months	75 mg
Children 1 – 3 years	80 mg
Children 4 – 8 years	130 mg
Children 9 – 13 years	240 mg
Children 14 – 18 years	
Girls	360 mg
Boys	410 mg
19 – 30 years	
Women	310 mg
Men	400 mg
31 years and older	
Women	320 mg
Men	420 mg

Pregnant women	
19 – 30 years	350 mg
31 years and older	360 mg
Breastfeeding women	
19 – 30 years	310 mg
31 years and older	320 mg

Leafy greens, legumes, nuts, seeds, fish and whole grains are the best and healthiest sources of magnesium. The following list is designed to give you a general indication of some healthy food items and their respective magnesium contents.

FOOD ITEM (How much?) = MAGNESIUM CONTENT (in mg)

- Beans (3/4 cup) = 58 – 89
- Bran flakes cereal (30 g) = 49 – 69
- Potato with skin (1 medium potato) = 47 – 52
- Avocado (1 cup) = 44
- Milk (1 cup) = 24 – 27
- Yogurt (8 oz.) = 42
- Banana (1 medium banana) = 32
- Apple (1 medium apple) = 9
- Spinach (1/2 cup) = 83
- Broccoli (1/2 cup) = 12
- All Bran cereal (1/3 cup) = 83 – 111
- Pumpkin seeds (1/4 cup) = 307
- Sunflower seeds (1/4 cup) = 129

- Almonds (1/4 cup) = 88 – 109

Because of all the above reasons, maintaining a healthy electrolyte balance is central to your health and blood pressure. Researchers have shown that diets low in sodium and rich in potassium, calcium and magnesium, play a crucial role in blood pressure control. The DASH diet outlined in *Section 3, subsection 2 and 3* provides adequate amounts calcium and magnesium through fruits, vegetables, fat-free and low-fat dairy products.

Section 5: Conclusion

I would like to take this opportunity to thank you for downloading this book. I hope you now have a solid understanding of blood pressure, how to reduce your blood pressure without medications, and that you are equipped with the knowledge to put you on the path to lifelong health and wellness!

My final piece of advice – every little step helps! Take small and gradual steps that will help you to continuously progress. Most importantly, stay optimistic, motivated, and focused on your goal! Improving your health and lowering your blood pressure is a lifelong investment in your wellbeing.

I sincerely wish you the best of luck in your journey.

Best wishes,

Eva Coleman

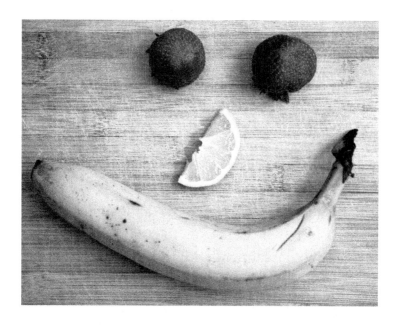

Bonus 1: Blood Pressure Solutions: 5 Secret Weapons!

Blood Pressure Solution Secret 1: Tomato Extract

Tomato extract contains carotenoids such as lycopene, beta carotene, and vitamin E. These are known to be effective antioxidants that can slow down the development of atherosclerosis. Researchers from the university of Negev in Israel have shown treatment with tomato extract rich in antioxidants to reduce blood pressure in patients with stage 1 hypertension. In a small study, a group of people with stage 1 high blood pressure took 250 milligrams of tomato extract, containing 15 milligrams of lycopene, daily for eight weeks. The daily intake of tomato extract was linked to a drop of 10 points in systolic blood pressure and a drop of 4 points in diastolic blood pressure.

Although researchers are currently unsure as to the exact way in which the consumption of tomato extract or regular tomatoes can help lower blood pressure, lycopene is credited with the blood pressure-lowering effect. Further research is needed to confirm this and to make definitive recommendations. Despite this, getting enough lycopene in your diet is definitely good for the health of your heart. The antioxidant can be found in red fruits such as tomato extract, tomatoes, pink grapefruit and watermelon. Please note however that tomato extract is not a substitute for adopting healthy lifestyle recommendations or for following your doctor's recommendations.

Blood Pressure Solution Secret 2: Grape Seed Extract

Grape seed extract has also shown to have a blood pressure-lowering effect. A study from the University of California, Davis, has evaluated the ability of grape seed extract to lower blood pressure in individuals with hypertension. The subjects across the board experienced an average drop of 12 points in their systolic blood pressure and an average reduction of 8 points in their diastolic blood pressure. The scientists from the university concluded grape seed extract to be a safe way to reduce blood pressure in people with hypertension. The extract is thought to have a blood pressure-lowering effect through helping arteries dilate.

If you are thinking of taking grape seed extract to treat hypertension, it is nevertheless strongly advised to consult with your doctor at first. Lastly, it is important to note that the above study was funded by Polyphenolics Inc., a producer of grape seed extract.

Blood Pressure Solution Secret 5: Cocoa

Although officially unconfirmed, cocoa is thought to be an important mediator that has beneficial effects on blood pressure, platelet and vascular function, and insulin resistance.

Researchers from the Cochrane Library have found that dark chocolate and cocoa have had slight blood pressure-lowering effects. This is because these foods both contain flavanols that boost nitrous oxide production in the body that causes arteries to relax and open.

Cocoa flavanols is therefore thought to help lower blood pressure by increasing flow-mediated vasodilation as well as by improving blood cholesterol. Vasodilation is the dilatation of blood vessels that has the effect of lowering blood pressure.

Long-term trials are still needed to investigate the definite effect of cocoa on cardiovascular health. Chocolate and cocoa products that are rich in flavanol have nevertheless shown to lower blood pressure by as much as 2 – 3 mm Hg in the short-term. It is important to note however, that only high-quality cocoa or dark chocolate count.

Blood Pressure Solution Secret 4: L-arginine

L-arginine is an amino acid that, with mixed results, has shown to lower blood pressure in some people. The amino acid is available as a supplement but is also found in foods such as whole grains, beans, dairy products, soy, nuts, fish and red meat. L-arginine converts to nitric oxide which can help lower blood pressure by opening and relaxing arteries.

Most people will naturally produce all the L-arginine they need. Larger studies are needed before we can positively determine whether or not L-arginine can reliably and safely lower blood pressure.

L-arginine supplements can interact with other medications, including some high blood pressure medications and some health conditions. Because of this, it is crucial to always talk to your physician before taking any nutritional or herbal supplements. This is particularly important if you are currently on medications or are undergoing a different health therapy.

Blood Pressure Solution Secret 5: Pycnogenol

Pycnogenol is an antioxidant supplement derived from the pine bark. Research that appeared in the journal *Life Sciences* suggests that pycnogenol can help people control their blood pressure as well as reduce their dependence on blood pressure medications. In a study with people with high blood pressure who have been prescribed blood pressure medication, the supplement has shown to lower their dependency on such medications. After 12 weeks, those with the antioxidant supplement were able to keep their blood pressure within the normal range with a 15-milligram dose of blood pressure medication compared to the average 21.6-milligram dose of medication in those who took the placebo.

Pycnogenol is thought to have antioxidant effects, stimulate the immune system, and contain substances that improve blood flow.

As with other supplements, due to potential adverse effects as well as interactions with other medications, it is strongly advised to speak to your doctor before taking pycnogenol. Caution and an initial consultation with your doctor is of utmost important - particularly with regards to children, pregnant women, and people with diabetes or other health complications.

Bonus 2: Juicing Recipes for Heart Health

Juicing is an incredibly healthy habit to get into and in this section I will share some of my favorite recipes with you. It is a good way to use up overripe fruit and a fun way to make sure you get your daily fix of healthy fruits! Note however that this is not a recommendation for juice fasting, and the recipes listed are not a substitute for the DASH diet. If you do decide to juice fast, always talk to your doctor first.

Preparation for smoothies couldn't be easier – just add all ingredients into a blender and blend until smooth!

Breakfast Smoothie

Ingredients:

- 1 cup frozen mixed berries
- 1 medium banana
- 1 medium pear
- 1 scoop Profibe
- 2 ounces frozen orange juice concentrate
- 4 oz. egg substitute
- 8 oz. nonfat or low fat milk or almond milk
- 8 oz. water or orange juice

Summer Medley

Ingredients:

- 2 cups cantaloupe melon chunks
- 2 cups honeydew melon chunks
- 2 cups seedless watermelon chunks
- 2 tablespoons honey
- 8 oz. orange juice

Banana Blueberry Detox

Ingredients:

- 1 – 2 cups fresh or frozen blueberries
- 1 scoop Profibe
- 2 medium bananas
- 2 oz. frozen red grape juice concentrate
- 4 oz. egg substitute
- 8 oz. nonfat or low-fat milk or almond milk
- 8 oz. water

Strawberry-Banana Smoothie with Cocoa

Ingredients:

- 1 medium banana

- 1 scoop Profibe
- 2 cups fresh or frozen strawberries
- 2 oz. frozen white grape juice
- 2 tablespoons cocoa powder
- 4 oz. egg substitute
- 8 oz. nonfat or low-fat milk or almond milk
- 8 oz. water

Fruit Punch with A Smooth Twist

Ingredients:

- 1 medium banana
- 1 medium mango or 1 cup of frozen raspberries
- 1 scoop Profibe
- 1 tablespoon honey
- 2 tablespoons cocoa powder
- 4 oz. egg substitute
- 8 oz. nonfat or low-fat milk or almond milk
- 8 oz. water

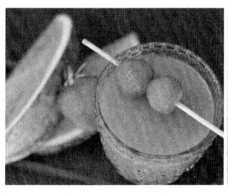 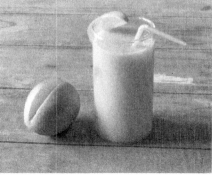

Eva Coleman

Bonus 3: Recipes for Healthy Blood Pressure

Salads

Three-Bean Salad

Ingredients:

- 1 teaspoon salt
- 1 teaspoon pepper
- 16 oz. can cut green beans, drained and rinsed
- 16 oz. can garbanzo beans, drained and rinsed
- 16 oz. can kidney beans, drained and rinsed
- 1/2 cup canola oil
- 1/2 cup red onions, chopped
- 1/2 cherry tomatoes, sliced in half
- 3/4 cup red or white wine vinegar
- 2 tablespoons of lemon juice

Instructions:

1. Remember to drain and rinse all of the canned beans to remove any excess sodium.
2. Chop the red onions and cherry tomatoes and add to a large bowl with all the other ingredients.
3. Refrigerate the bowl for a few hours or overnight and leave to develop a rich flavor.
4. Stir and enjoy!

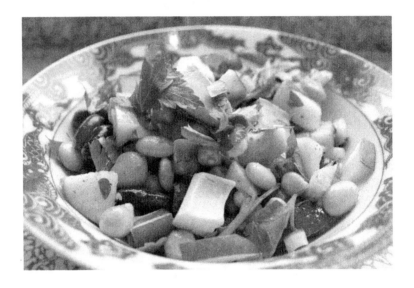

Sweet Potato Salad

Ingredients:

- 2 large sweet potatoes with skin
- 1 cup celery (4 to 5 stalks), diced
- 1 cup apples, diced
- 1/3 cup walnuts, chopped
- 2 tablespoons lemon juice
- Salt (optional)
- Low-fat mayonnaise

Instructions:

1. Cut the sweet potatoes into small chunks and leave the skin on to preserve the nutrients and fiber. Boil it in water until tender. Feel free to add a pinch of salt to the water.

2. Prepare all the other ingredients and mix in a large bowl with the sweet potatoes.

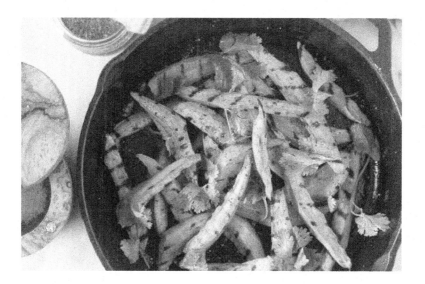

Soups

Creamy Vegetable Soup

Ingredients:

- 1 cup low-fat sour cream

- 1/2 teaspoon ground white pepper
- 1/2 teaspoon tarragon
- 1/2 teaspoon thyme
- 2 bay leaves
- 4 cups cauliflower, broccoli florets, asparagus, carrots, or root vegetables
- 4 cups low-sodium vegetable, chicken, or beef broth

Instructions:

1. Place the sour cream to the side and put all other ingredients into a large pot.
2. Bring the pot to boil, then simmer, and cook down all vegetables until they have a mushy consistency.
3. Leave the soup to cool.
4. Remove the bay leaves and blend the rest in a food processor or blender
5. Put the soup back into the pot, blend in the sour cream and heat it up.

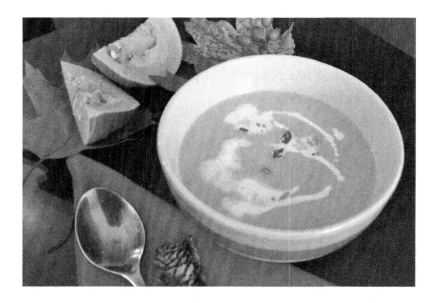

Minestrone Soup

Ingredients:

- 1 can low-sodium whole Italian tomatoes, cut into chunks
- 1 tablespoon tomato paste
- 1 can white or kidney beans, drained and rinsed
- 1 medium onion, minced
- 1 scallion or spring onion, minced
- 1 package frozen spinach
- 1/2 cup frozen peas
- 1/2 tablespoon Italian seasoning
- 1/2 teaspoon fresh ground black pepper
- 2 bay leaves
- 2 celery stalks, diced

- 2 medium carrots, peeled and diced
- 2 quarts of low-sodium vegetable or chicken broth
- 2 sweet or red potatoes, unpeeled and diced
- 2 zucchinis, diced
- 2 teaspoons olive oil
- 3 tablespoons parsley or broad leaf, chopped
- 4 oz. elbow macaroni pasta
- Salt (optional)

Instructions:

1. Fry the onions and scallion in a large pot in olive oil until brown.
2. Add the carrots to the pot and fry for 2 – 5 minutes.
3. Put the macaroni, spinach, tomatoes, peas and parsley to the side.
4. Add all other ingredients to the pot. Bring to boil, then lower the heat and leave to simmer for 1 hour.
5. Add the macaroni, spinach, tomatoes, peas and parsley to the soup and simmer for another 10 minutes.
6. Add salt and pepper. If you wish, you can leave the soup overnight and heat it up again the next day for a richer flavor.

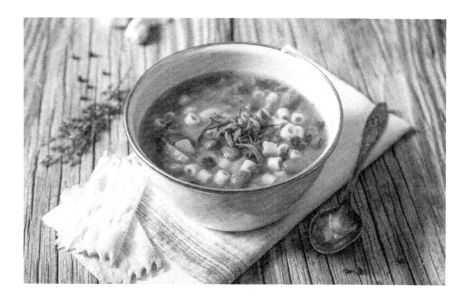

Other Main Dishes

<u>Polenta with Mediterranean Vegetables</u>

Ingredients:

- 1 ½ cups coarse polenta (corn grits)
- 1 small eggplant, peeled and diced
- 1 small green zucchini, diced
- 1 small yellow zucchini, diced
- 1 sweet red pepper, seeded, cored and cut into small chunks
- 1/4 teaspoon black pepper
- 10 oz. frozen spinach, thawed
- 10 ripe olives, chopped

- 2 ½ tablespoons olive oil
- 2 plum tomatoes, sliced
- 2 teaspoons of trans-free margarine
- 2 teaspoons oregano
- 6 cups water
- 6 dry-packed sun-dried tomatoes, soaked in water, drained and chopped
- 6 medium mushrooms, sliced

Instructions:

1. Prepare the red pepper, eggplant, mushrooms and zucchini and brush with 1 tablespoon of olive oil. Broil under low heat in the grill, turn upside down as need until tender and golden brown.
2. Preheat the oven to 350 degrees Fahrenheit.
3. Coat your oven dish with cooking spray or a thin layer of trans-free margarine and place to the side.
4. Drain your spinach and place to the side.
5. Bring water to boil in a medium saucepan. Reduce the heat and gradually whisk in the polenta. Stir and cook for 5 minutes. Slowly add in the margarine, seasoning and black pepper.
6. Spread the polenta on the base of your oven dish. Place the dish inside the oven and leave to bake for 10 minutes.
7. After 10 minutes, remove the dish from the oven and top the polenta with the drained spinach. Also add a second layer of chopped sun-dried tomatoes, sliced tomatoes and olives. Add a third layer with some

roasted vegetables and sprinkle some oregano and black pepper over the entire dish.

8. Return to the oven for another 10 minutes.

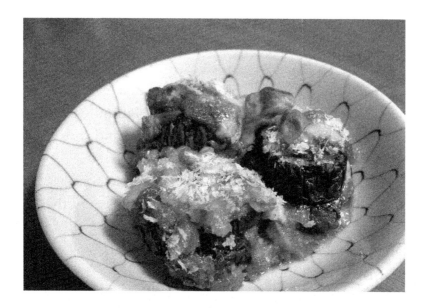

Quinoa Risotto with Rocket Salad and Parmesan

Ingredients:

- 1 tablespoon olive oil
- 1 garlic clove, minced
- 1 cup quinoa, well rinsed
- 2 cups washed rocket salad
- 1 small carrot, peeled and finely shredded
- 1/2 yellow onion, chopped
- 1/2 cup thinly sliced fresh shiitake mushrooms

- 1/2 teaspoon salt
- 2 1/4 cups low-sodium vegetable stock or broth
- 1/4 cup grated Parmesan cheese
- 1/4 teaspoon ground black pepper

Instructions:

1. Heat the olive oil to medium heat in a large saucepan. Add the onion and fry for around 4 minutes until soft.
2. Add the quinoa and garlic to the pan and cook for around 1 minute.
3. Add the stock to the pan and bring it to boil.
4. Leave to simmer for around 12 minutes until the quinoa begins to tender.
5. Add the mushrooms and carrot to the risotto and simmer for another 2 minutes.
6. Remove from the heat, stir in the cheese and add the rocket salad. Add salt and pepper and serve.

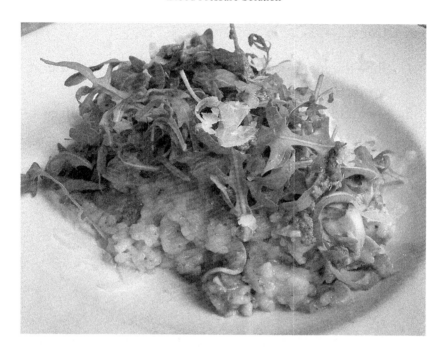

Desserts

Mango and Sticky rice

Ingredients:

- 1 large mango, peeled and sliced
- 2 cups of sticky rice, cooked in low-fat coconut milk or half water, half coconut milk
- Sesame seeds (optional)

Instructions:

1. Slice the mangoes and arrange on a plate with the warm rice.
2. Sprinkle some sesame seeds over the mango slices.
3. Enjoy!

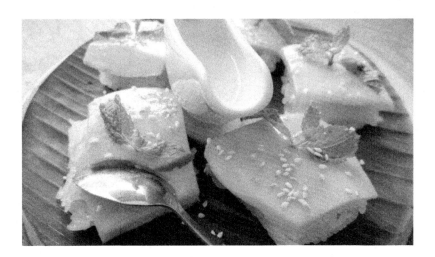

Banana Split

Ingredients:

- 2 bananas, sliced lengthwise
- Low-fat vanilla ice cream
- Walnuts, diced (optional)
- Coconut flakes (optional)
- Melted dark chocolate (optional)

Instructions:

1. Slice the bananas lengthwise and arrange on a dessert plate with the ice cream.
2. Sprinkle some coconut flakes or walnuts or create melted chocolate zigzag over the bananas and ice cream.
3. Enjoy!

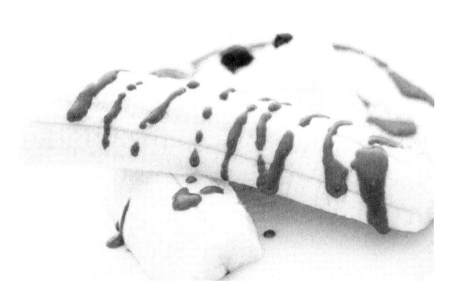

Free Blood Pressure Solution Audiobook

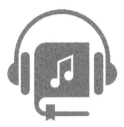

Visit Blood-Pressure-Solutions.com to get instant access to your free audio program!

CPSIA information can be obtained
at www.ICGtesting.com
Printed in the USA
LVOW13s1846291117
558026LV00014B/1092/P